Virtual Clinical Excursions—Pediatrics

for

James, Ashwill, and Droske:

Nursing Care of Children: Principles & Practice
Second Edition

prepared by

Janet T. Ihlenfeld, RN, PhD
Professor
Department of Nursing
D'Youville College
Buffalo, New York

Virtual Clinical Excursions Author and Software Design

Jay Shiro Tashiro, PhD, RN
Director of Systems Design
Wolfsong Informatics
Tucson, Arizona

Ellen Sullins, PhD
Director of Research
Wolfsong Informatics
Tucson, Arizona

Gina Long, RN, DNSc
Assistant Professor, Department of Nursing
College of Health Professions
Northern Arizona University
Flagstaff, Arizona

Software Development

Michael Kelly
Developer and Programmer
Michael M. Kelly and Associates
Flagstaff, Arizona

SAUNDERS
An Imprint of Elsevier Science
Philadelphia   London   New York   St. Louis   Sydney   Toronto

SAUNDERS, INC.
The Curtis Center
Independence Square West
Philadelphia, Pennsylvania 19106-3399

Virtual Clinical Excursions for James, Ashwill, and Droske:
Nursing Care of Children: Principles & Practice, Second Edition
Copyright © 2003, Saunders, Inc. All rights reserved.

Notice

Pharmacology is an ever-changing field. Standard safety precautions must be followed, but as new research and clinical experience broaden our knowledge, changes in treatment and drug therapy may become necessary or appropriate. Readers are advised to check the most current product information provided by the manufacturer of each drug to be administered to verify the recommended dose, the method and duration of administration, and contraindications. It is the responsibility of the licensed prescriber, relying on experience and knowledge of the patient, to determine dosages and the best treatment for each individual patient. Neither the publisher nor the editor assumes any liability for any injury and/or damage to persons or property arising from this publication.

The Publisher

First Edition 2003.

Executive Vice President, Nursing & Health Professions: Sally Schrefer
Editor, Nursing: Tom Wilhelm
Senior Developmental Editor: Jeff Downing
Project Manager: Gayle May
Designer: Wordbench
Cover Art: Jyotika Schrof

Printed in the United States of America

Last digit is the print number: 9   8   7   6   5   4   3   2   1

Workbook
prepared by

Janet T. Ihlenfeld, RN, PhD
Professor
Department of Nursing
D'Youville College
Buffalo, New York

Textbook

Susan Rowen James, RN, MSN
Associate Professor
Division of Nursing Studies
Curry College
Milton, Massachusetts

Jean Weiler Ashwill, RN, MSN
Director
Center for Continuing Nursing Education
School of Nursing
The University of Texas at Arlington
Arlington, Texas

Susan Colvert Droske, RN, MSN, CPN
Associate Professor of Nursing
Texarkana College
Texarkana, Texas

Dedication

This book is dedicated to seekers of knowledge everywhere.

Janet T. Ihlenfeld

Contents

Getting Started

GETTING SET UP

◼ MINIMUM SYSTEM REQUIREMENTS

Virtual Clinical Excursions—Pediatrics is a hybrid CD, so it runs on both Macintosh and Windows platforms. To use *Virtual Clinical Excursions—Pediatrics*, you will need one of the following systems:

- **Windows™**

  Windows XP, 2000, 98, 95, NT 4.0
  IBM-compatible computer
  Pentium II processor (or equivalent)
  300 MHz
  96 MB (minimum) of RAM
  800 × 600 screen size
  Thousands of colors
  100 MB hard drive space
  12× CD-ROM drive
  Soundblaster 16 soundcard compatibility
  Stereo speakers or headphones

- **Macintosh®**

  MAC OS 9.04
  Apple Power PC G3
  300 MHz
  96 MB (minimum) of RAM
  800 × 600 screen size
  Thousands of colors
  100 MB hard drive space
  12× CD-ROM drive
  Stereo speakers or headphones

Note: *Virtual Clinical Excursions—Pediatrics* is not designed to function at a 256-color depth. You may need to access the Control Panel on your computer and adjust the Display setting. See specific instructions for this in How to Adjust Your Monitor's Settings on p. 2 of this workbook.

■ INSTALLING *VIRTUAL CLINICAL EXCURSIONS—PEDIATRICS*

Virtual Clinical Excursions—Pediatrics is designed to run from a set of files installed on your hard drive and a CD inserted in your CD-ROM drive. Minimal installation is required.

- **Windows™**

  1. Start Microsoft Windows and insert *Virtual Clinical Excursions—Pediatrics* **Disk 1 (Installation)** in the CD-ROM drive.
  2. Click the **Start** icon on the taskbar and select the **Run** option.
  3. Type d:\setup.exe (where "d:\" is your CD-ROM drive) and press **OK**.
  4. Follow the on-screen instructions for installation.
  5. Remove *Virtual Clinical Excursions—Pediatrics* **Disk 1 (Installation)** from your CD-ROM drive.
  6. Restart your computer.

- **Macintosh®**

  1. Insert *Virtual Clinical Excursions—Pediatrics* **Disk 1 (Installation)** in the CD-ROM drive. The disk icon will appear on your desktop.
  2. Double-click on the disk icon.
  3. Double-click on the icon **Install Virtual Clinical Excursions**.
  4. Follow the on-screen instructions for installation.
  5. Remove *Virtual Clinical Excursions—Pediatrics* **Disk 1 (Installation)** from your CD-ROM drive.
  6. Restart your computer.

■ HOW TO ADJUST YOUR MONITOR'S SETTINGS (WINDOWS™ ONLY)

- **Windows 95/98/SE/ME/2000**

  1. Click the **Start** button and go to **Settings** on the pop-up menu. Click on **Control Panel**.
  2. When the Control Panel window opens, double-click on the **Display** icon.
  3. This opens the Display Properties window. Click on the **Settings** tab (on the top right). Below the image of the monitor, you will find the settings for color quality and screen resolution. Change this to **High Color (16 bit)** by selecting it from the drop down menu. On the right is the Desktop area. Click and hold down on the slider button and move it to 800 by 600 pixels. Now click **OK**.
  4. If Windows™ asks you to confirm the change, click **OK**. Your screen will resize and Windows™ may again ask you whether you want to keep these new settings. Click **Yes**.

- **Windows XP**

  1. Click the **Start** button; then click **Control Panel** on the pop-up menu.
  2. Click **Display**. If Display does not appear, click **Switch to Classic View**; then click on **Display** icon.
  3. From the Display Properties dialog box, select the **Settings** tab.
  4. Under Screen Resolution, click and drag the sliding bar to adjust the Desktop size to 800 x 600.
  5. Under Color Quality, choose High or Highest.
  6. Click **Apply**. If you approve of the new settings, click **Yes**.

■ HOW TO USE DISK 2 (PATIENTS' DISK)

- **Windows™**

  When you want to work with any of the five patients in the virtual hospital, follow these steps:

  1. Insert *Virtual Clinical Excursions—Pediatrics* **Disk 2 (Patients' Disk)** into your CD-ROM drive.
  2. Double-click on the icon **Shortcut to VCE Pediatrics**, which can be found on your desktop. This will load and run the program.

- **Macintosh®**

  When you want to work with any of the five patients in the virtual hospital, follow these steps:

  1. Insert *Virtual Clinical Excursions—Pediatrics* **Disk 2 (Patients' Disk)** into your CD-ROM drive.
  2. Double-click on the icon **Shortcut to VCE Pediatrics**, which can be found on your desktop. This will load and run the program.

■ QUALITY OF VISUALS, SPEED, AND COMMON PROBLEMS

Virtual Clinical Excursions—Pediatrics uses the Apple QuickTime media layer system. This includes QuickTime Video and QuickTime VR Video, which allow for high-quality graphics and digital video. The graphics seen in the *Virtual Clinical Excursions—Pediatrics* courseware should be of high quality with good color. If the movies and graphics appear blocky or grainy, check to see whether your video card is set to "thousands of colors."

Note: Virtual Clinical Excursions—Pediatrics is not designed to function at a 256-color depth. To adjust your monitor's settings, see instructions on p. 2.

The system should respond quickly and smoothly. In particular, you should not see any jerky motions or experience unusual delays as you move through the virtual hospital settings, interact with patients, or access information resources. If you notice slow, jerky, or delayed software responses, it may mean that your particular system requires additional RAM, your processor does not meet the basic requirements, or your hard drive is full or too fragmented. If the videos appear banded or subject to "breakup," you may need to find an updated video driver for the computer's video card. Please consult the manufacturer of the video card or computer for additional video drivers for your machine.

If you are experiencing misplacement of text or cursors in the Electronic Patient Record (EPR), it is likely that your computer operating system has enabled font smoothing. Please turn font smoothing off by following these instructions:

- **Windows™**

  From the Control Panel window select **Display** and then select the **Effects** tab. Make sure the "Smooth Edges of Screen Fonts" is unselected.

- **Macintosh®**

  From the desktop, click on the **Apple** icon in the upper left corner. From the drop-down menu, select **Control Panel**; then select **Appearance**. Click on the **Fonts** tab and make sure the selection box next to "Smooth all fonts on screen" is unselected.

Virtual Clinical Excursions—Pediatrics uses the Adobe Acrobat Reader version 5 to display information in certain places in the simulation. If you cannot see any information when accessing the Charts, Medication Administration Record (MAR), or Kardex, it is likely that the Adobe Acrobat Reader was not installed properly when you installed *Virtual Clinical Excursions—Pediatrics*. To remedy this, you can manually install the Acrobat Reader from the *Virtual Clinical Excursions—Pediatrics* **Disk 1 (Installation)**. Double-click the **Adobe Acrobat Reader** installer (ar505enu.exe) on the disk and follow the on-screen instructions. Once the installer has finished installing the Acrobat Reader, restart your computer and then resume your use of *Virtual Clinical Excursions—Pediatrics*.

■ TECHNICAL SUPPORT

Technical support for this product is available at no charge by calling the Technical Support Hotline between 9 a.m. and 5 p.m. (Central Time), Monday through Friday. Inside the United States, call 1-800-692-9010. Outside the United States, call 314-872-8370.

Trademarks: Windows™ is a registered trademark.

A QUICK TOUR

Welcome to *Virtual Clinical Excursions—Pediatrics*, a virtual hospital setting in which you can work with seven patient simulations and also learn to access and evaluate the health information resources that are essential for high-quality patient care. As you use this workbook and software, you will find that the exercises guide you to conduct assessments, to review patient records, and to plan care for your patients.

Canyon View Regional Medical Center, is a multistory teaching hospital with a Well-Child Clinic, Pediatric Floor, Surgery Department, Intensive Care Unit, and a Medical-Surgical Floor with a Telemetry Unit. You will have access to the pediatric patients within the Well-Child Clinic and Pediatric Floor. One patient will also spend time in the Surgery Department, where you can follow him through a perioperative experience.

Although each floor plan in the medical center is different, each is based on a realistic hospital architecture modeled from a composite of several hospital settings. All floors have:

- A Nurses' Station
- Patients, seen either in examination areas or in their inpatient rooms
- Patient records (*Note*: The Well-Child Clinic keeps only one type of patient record—the Chart. However, on the Pediatric Floor and in the Surgery Department, patient records are kept in several formats—the Chart, Kardex plan of care, Medication Administration Record, and Electronic Patient Record.)

■ BEFORE YOU START

When you use *Virtual Clinical Excursions—Pediatrics*, make sure you have your textbook nearby to consult topic areas as needed. Also remember that you must have your Patients' Disk to run the simulations. If you have not already installed your *VCE-Pediatrics* software, do so now by following the steps outlined in **Getting Set Up** at the beginning of this workbook.

■ ENTERING THE HOSPITAL AND SELECTING A CLINICAL ROTATION

To begin your tour of Canyon View Regional Medical Center, insert your *Virtual Clinical Excursions—Pediatrics* Patients' Disk and double-click on the desktop icon **Shortcut to VCE Pediatrics.** Wait for the hospital entrance screen to appear (see below). This is your signal that the program is ready to run. Your first task is to get to the unit where you will be caring for patients and to let someone know when you arrive at the unit. As in any multistory hospital, you will enter the hospital lobby area, take an elevator to your assigned unit, and sign in at the Nurses' Station.

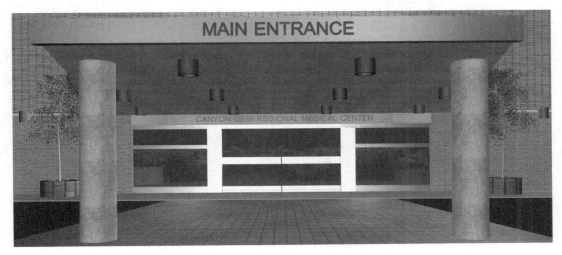

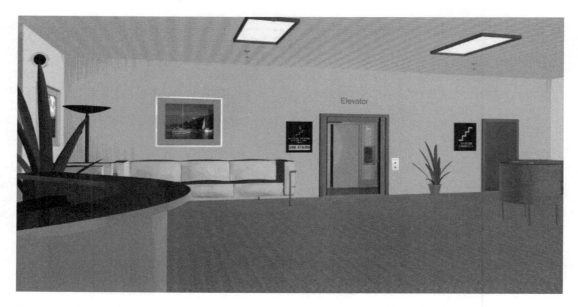

Let's practice getting to your unit in Canyon View Regional Medical Center by following this sequence:

- Click on the hospital entrance door and you will find yourself in the hospital lobby on the first floor (see above).
- Across the lobby, you will see an elevator with a blinking red light. Click on the open doorway and you will be transported into the elevator (see below).
- Now click on the panel on the right side of the doorway. The panel will expand to reveal buttons that allow you to go to the other floors of the hospital.
- Slowly run your cursor across the buttons to familiarize yourself with the different floors and units of the hospital.

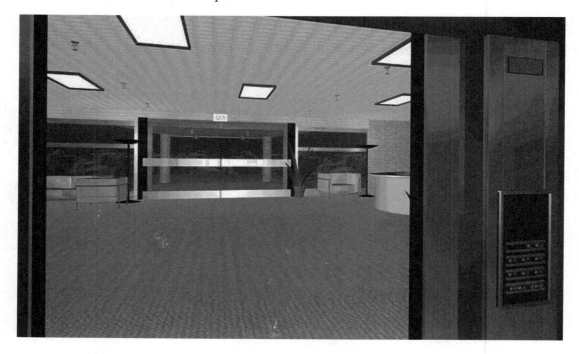

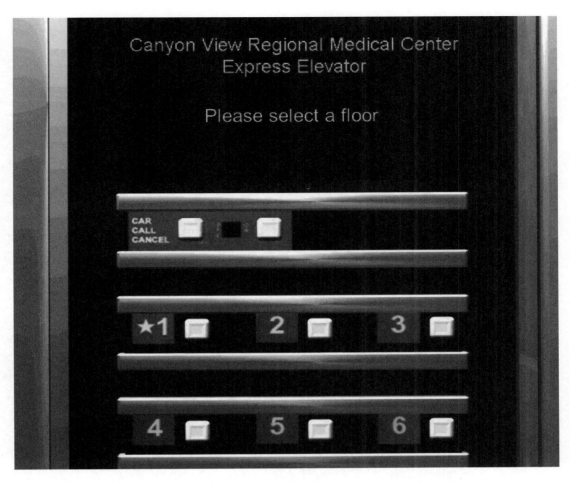

You are currently in a pediatric rotation, so you will not be able to visit the Intensive Care Unit or Medical-Surgical/Telemetry Floor. However, you can work with three children in the Well-Child Clinic, three on the Pediatric Floor, and one who spends time on the Pediatric Floor and in the Surgery Department.

Now, go to Pediatrics and sign in for patient care. To do this:

- Click on the button for the Pediatric Floor (Floor 3).
- The elevator takes you to Floor 3 and opens onto a virtual Pediatric Unit with a Nurses' Station in the center and rooms arranged around the Nurses' Station.
- Click on the **Nurses' Station** and you will be transported inside the station, behind its counter.
- If you click and hold down your mouse button, you can get a 360° view of the Pediatric Floor by dragging your mouse to the left or right. Practice dragging left and right, then up and down, to get a complete view of the Nurses' Station and the Pediatric Floor.
- Take a few minutes to familiarize yourself with the Nurses' Station. First, find the computer with the word **Login** on its screen. This is the Supervisor's Computer, which allows you to select a patient to work with. Now click and drag your mouse to the right or left until you see another computer. This computer allows you to access the **Electronic Patient Records (EPR)** system. Continue browsing around the Nurses' Station until you have found the patient Charts, the Kardex plan of care notebooks, and the Medication Administration Record (MAR).

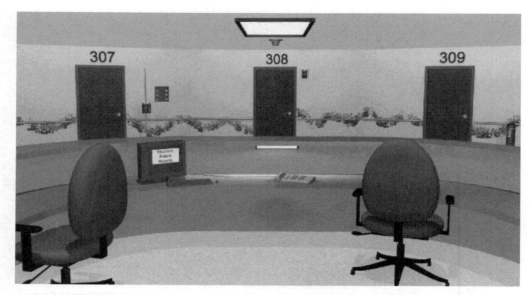

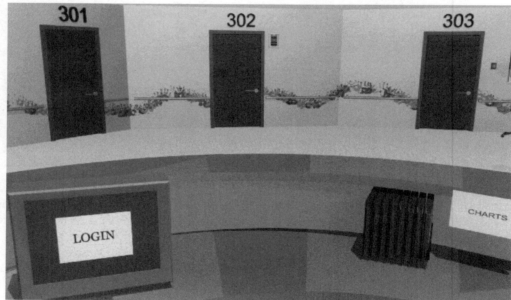

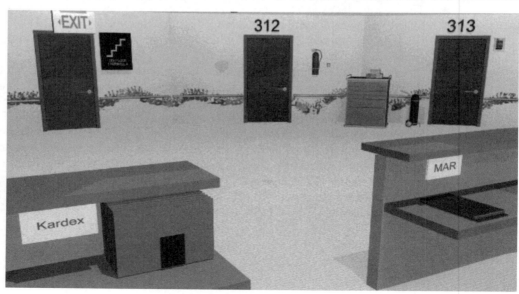

■ WORKING WITH PATIENTS

The Pediatric Floor can be visited from 0700 to 1500, but you can see only one patient at a time and only in specified blocks of time. We call these blocks *periods of care*. In any of the Pediatric Floor scenarios, you can select a patient and a period of care by accessing the Supervisor's (Login) Computer. Double-click on this computer to open the sign-in screen, which contains a box with instructions. Click the **Login** button and you will see a screen that lists the patients on this floor and the periods of care in which you can visit and work with them. Again, only one patient can be selected at a time. When you have completed a period of care with one patient, you can select another period of care for that patient or select another pediatric patient.

Note: During a patient simulation you may receive an on-screen message informing you that the current period of care has ended. If this occurs and you have not yet completed the assigned activities (or if you want to review part of the simulation), simply return to the Supervisor's Computer and sign in again for the same patient and period of care.

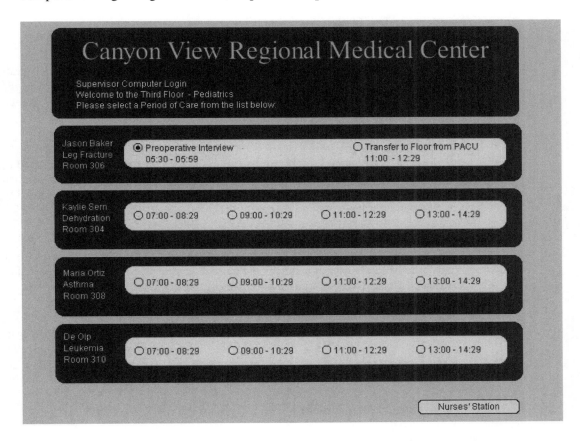

You can choose any of the four patients on this floor (but only one at a time). When you choose a patient, you must also select a period of care. Three of the patients (De Olp, Kaylie Sern, and Maria Ortiz) can be seen during the following four periods of care: 0700–0829, 0900–1029, 1100–1229, and 1300–1429. The fourth patient, Jason Baker, can be seen on the Pediatric Floor from 0500 to 0529 for a preoperative interview. He then goes to the Surgery Department for preoperative care, surgery, and a period in the PACU (from 0630 to 1029). Jason returns to the Pediatric Floor at 1100, after leaving PACU. You can then see him on the Pediatric Floor from 1100 to 1229. (*Note:* The process of selecting patients is basically the same on all floors of Canyon View Regional Medical Center, although the available periods of care in the Well-Child Clinic and the Surgery Department are different from those on the Pediatric Floor. You will observe this when you visit the other floors.) Take a few minutes now to become acquainted with all the patients you will work with.

■ PATIENT LIST

◆ Floor 2: Well-Child Clinic

- Paul Parker (Room 202)
  Paul is a 24-month-old child visiting for a routine well-child examination. He has a history of ear infections. He is accompanied by his mother.

- Sherrie Bedonie (Room 204)
  Sherrie, a 48-month-old child, has come to the clinic for a routine well-child visit. Sherrie's mother is with her throughout the examination.

- Matthew Brown (Room 205)
  Matthew is a 10-month-old child. He and his father have come to the clinic for a well-child examination.

◆ Floor 3: Pediatric Floor

- Kaylie Sern (Room 304)
  Kaylie is a 3-year-old brought to the Emergency Department by her foster mother. She has had a fever and poor appetite for the past 48 hours. Kaylie has a primary diagnosis of dehydration and a secondary diagnosis of acute bilateral otitis media. She was admitted for observation and rehydration.

- Jason Baker (Room 306)
  Jason is a 14-year-old brought to the Emergency Department with a fractured right tibia and fibula, as well as a possible closed head injury. Jason also has type 1 diabetes mellitus, managed with insulin injections. He has been scheduled for surgical repair of his lower right leg.

- Maria Ortiz (Room 308)
  Maria is an 8-year-old child who was admitted from the Emergency Department with an acute exacerbation of asthma. She has a 2-year history of asthma. Past acute exacerbation have been treated with Prelone.

- De Olp (Room 310)
  De is a 6-year-old girl who entered the hospital 4 days ago. A bone marrow aspiration confirmed a diagnosis of acute lymphoblastic leukemia. She has had a lumbar puncture for assessment of cerebral spinal fluid, intrathecal chemotherapy, and placement of a Port-a-Cath for administering additional chemotherapy agents.

◆ Floor 4: Surgery Department

- Jason Baker
  Jason begins Tuesday on the Pediatric Floor (see Room 306 above). He is then transferred to the Surgery Department and undergoes surgical repair of his leg fracture. After a period in the Post-Anesthesia Care Unit (PACU), he is transferred back to the Pediatric Floor and into the same room he left earlier this morning.

▪ VISITING A PATIENT

Each time you sign in for a new patient and period of care, you enter the simulation at the start of that period of care. The simulations are constructed so that you can conduct a fairly complete assessment of your patient in the first 30 minutes of each period of care. However, after completing a general survey, you should begin to focus your assessments on specific areas. For example, you should not do a head-to-toe examination each time you come into a patient's room; instead you should select assessments that are appropriate for your patient's current condition and based on how that condition is changing. Just as in the real world, a patient's data will change through time as he or she improves or deteriorates. Even if a patient remains stable, there will be diurnal variations in physiology and these will be reflected in changes in assessment data.

As soon as you sign in to begin working with a patient, a clock appears to help you keep track of time. The clock, which operates in "real time," is located in the bottom left-hand corner of the screen when you are in the Nurses' Station and in the top right-hand corner when you are in a patient's room.

To become familiar with some of the learning resources in VCE, select Maria Ortiz and choose the 0700–0829 period of care. Then click on **Nurses' Station** in the lower right corner. This procedure selects the patient and time period for your shift and sends you to a brief Case Overview. The Case Overview begins with a short video in which your preceptor asks you to review a summary on this patient. Below the video screen is a button labeled **Assignment**. Click on this button to open a summary sheet that provides information about Maria and assigns tasks for you to complete when working with this patient.

After completing the Case Overview, click on **Nurses' Station** in the lower right corner of the screen. This will take you back to the Nurses' Station, where you can begin working with your patient. Remember three things:

- You must select a patient and period of care before any of that patient's simulation and data become available to you.
- Just as in the real world, the Nurses' Station is the base from which you can access patient records and from which you go onto the floor to visit a patient.
- Before you can see another patient or access another patient's record, you must go back to the Supervisor's (Login) Computer and follow the procedure to sign out from your current period of care.

Now that you have signed in for a patient, Maria Ortiz, you have several choices. You can enter Maria's room and work with your preceptor to assess your patient. You can review Maria's patient records, including her Chart, a Kardex plan of care, her active Medication Administration Record (MAR), and the Electronic Patient Record (EPR), all of which contain data that have been collected since Maria entered the hospital. You may know that some hospitals have only paper records; others have only electronic records. Canyon View Regional Medical Center, the *VCE* virtual hospital, has a combination of paper records (the patient's Chart, Kardex, MAR) and electronic records (the EPR).

Let's begin by becoming more familiar with the Nurses' Station screen. In the upper left hand corner, find a menu with these five buttons:

- Patient Care
- Planning Care
- Patient Records
- Case Conference
- Clinical Review

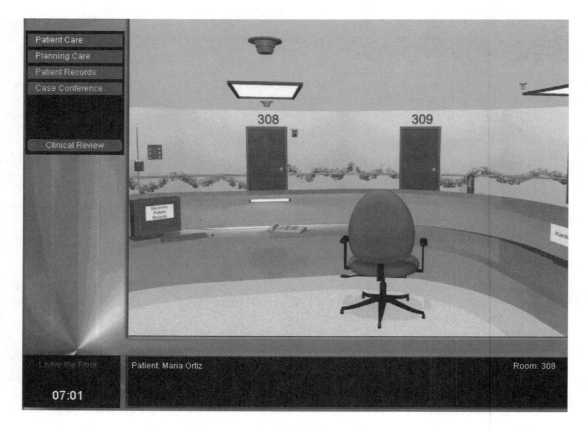

One at a time, single-click on these buttons to reveal drop-down menus with additional options for each item. First click on **Patient Care**. Two options are available for this item: **Case Overview** and **Data Collection**. You completed the Case Overview after signing in for Maria, but you can always go back to review it. For example, you might want to return there and click the **Assignment** button to review the summary of Maria's care up the start of your shift—or to remind yourself what tasks you have been asked to complete.

◆ **Data Collection**

To conduct an assessment of your patient, click **Patient Care** and then **Data Collection** from the drop-down menu. This will take you into a small anteroom (part of the patient's room) with a sink, laundry bin, and biohazards waste can. *Note:* You can also enter this anteroom by clicking on the outer door of Maria's room (Room 308). To visit your patient, complete these steps:

● First *wash your hands!* Click on the sink once to indicate you are beginning to wash. Click again to indicate you are finished washing.
● Now click on the curtain to the right of the sink and enter the patient's room.

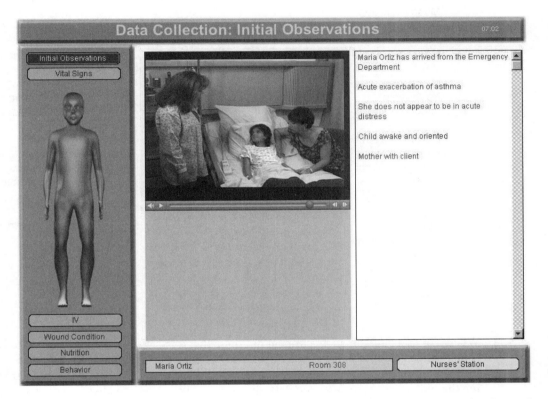

Once in the patient's room, your screen is equipped with various tools you can use for data collection. In the center of the screen, you will see a still frame of your patient. Along the left side of the screen are buttons and a body model that allow you to access learning activities in which your preceptor conducts different types of assessments. Try clicking on the buttons and different body parts. (Note that the body model rotates once your cursor touches it. As you move your cursor over the model, various body parts are highlighted in orange.)

What happened when you clicked on the buttons or body parts? Many of the buttons open options for additional assessments—these always appear below the picture of your patient. Likewise, clicking on a highlighted area of the body model opens options for additional assessments. The body model serves two purposes. First, it provides a way for you to develop a sense of what assessments and physiologic systems are associated with different areas of the human body. Second, it acts as a quick navigational tool that allows you to focus on certain types of assessments.

Note that the body model is a "generic" figure without specific sexual or racial characteristics. However, we encourage you to always think about your patients as unique individuals. The body model is simply a tool designed to help you develop assessment skills by body area and navigate quickly though the simulation's learning activities. Review the diagram below to become familiar with the available Data Collection buttons and the additional options that appear when you click each button and body area.

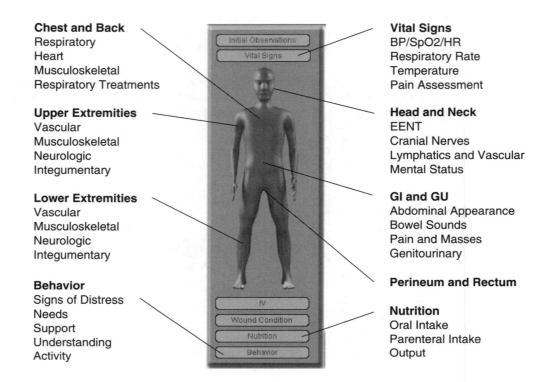

Chest and Back
Respiratory
Heart
Musculoskeletal
Respiratory Treatments

Upper Extremities
Vascular
Musculoskeletal
Neurologic
Integumentary

Lower Extremities
Vascular
Musculoskeletal
Neurologic
Integumentary

Behavior
Signs of Distress
Needs
Support
Understanding
Activity

Vital Signs
BP/SpO2/HR
Respiratory Rate
Temperature
Pain Assessment

Head and Neck
EENT
Cranial Nerves
Lymphatics and Vascular
Mental Status

GI and GU
Abdominal Appearance
Bowel Sounds
Pain and Masses
Genitourinary

Perineum and Rectum

Nutrition
Oral Intake
Parenteral Intake
Output

Whenever you click on an assessment button, either a video or still photo will be activated in the center of the screen. For some activities, data obtained during assessment are shown in a box to the right of that frame. For other assessment options, you must collect data yourself by observing the video—in these cases, no data appear in the box. You can always replay a video by simply reclicking the assessment button of the activity you wish to see again.

The *Virtual Clinical Excursions—Pediatrics* patient simulations were constructed by expert nurses to be as realistic as possible. As previously mentioned, the data for every patient change through time. During the first 30 minutes of a period of care, you will generally find that all assessment options will give you data on the patient. However, after that period, some assessments may no longer be a high priority for a patient. The expert nurses who created the patient simulations let you know when an assessment area is not a high priority by sending you a short message. These messages appear in the box on the right side of the screen, where data are normally listed. Some examples of messages you might receive include "Please rethink your priorities for assessment of this patient" and "Your assessment should be focused on other areas at this time."

To leave the patient's room, click on the **Nurses' Station** button in the bottom right-hand corner of the screen. Note that this takes you back through the anteroom, where you must wash your hands before leaving. Once you have washed your hands, click on the outer door to return to the Nurses' Station.

Now, let's review what you just learned and try a few quick exercises to get a sense of how the Data Collection learning activities become available to you. You are already signed in to care for Maria Ortiz, who entered the hospital this morning with acute exacerbations of asthma. Reenter her room from the Nurses' Station by clicking on **Patient Care** and then on **Data Collection**. You are now in the sink area of the patient's room, so wash your hands and click on the curtain to see the patient.

Start your patient care by collecting Maria's vital signs.

- Click on **Vital Signs**. Four assessment options will appear below the picture of the patient.
- Click on **BP/SpO$_2$/HR**. Watch the video as your preceptor measures blood pressure, oxygen saturation, and heart rate on a noninvasive multipurpose monitor. Record Maria's data for these attributes in the chart below.
- Now click on **Respiratory Rate**. This time, after a video plays, a "breathing" body model appears on the right. Measure Maria's respiratory rate by counting the respirations of the body model for the period of time your instructor recommends. Record your estimate of her respiratory rate.
- Next, click on **Temperature**. First, you will see your preceptor measuring Maria's temperature; then the thermometer reading appears in the frame to the right. Record her temperature.
- Finally, assess Maria's pain by clicking on **Pain Assessment**. Note your interpretation of Maria's pain. If she is in pain, record her pain level and characteristics.

Vital Signs	Time
Blood pressure	
SpO$_2$	
Heart rate	
Respiratory rate	
Temperature	
Pain rating	

Once you have collected Maria's vital signs, begin a chest examination. Point your cursor to the chest area of the body model. Click anywhere on the orange highlighted area. Four new options now appear below the picture of your patient.

- Click on **Respiratory**. Observe the video and note the data you obtain from this examination.
- Now click on **Respiratory Treatments**. How much oxygen is Maria receiving at this time?

You have now collected vital signs data and conducted a limited respiratory assessment of Maria, who was admitted with acute exacerbations of asthma. As previously mentioned, most of the assessments combine a video or still photo of the patient with data that are collected for the respective assessment. Other assessments simply provide a video, and you must collect data from the nurse-patient interaction. For example, many of the pain assessments consist of the nurse asking the patient to rate his or her pain and the patient responding with a rating. Some of the behavior assessments also require that you listen to the nurse-patient interaction and make a decision about the patient's condition, needs, or psychosocial attributes.

When you visit patients in the Well-Child Clinic and the Surgery Department, you will notice slightly different assessment options for some periods of care. However, the same types of interactions are always available. When you click on a button or area of the body model, you will be able to access a variety of patient assessments. If a video is shown, it can always be replayed by clicking on the assessment button.

■ HOW TO FIND AND ACCESS A PATIENT'S RECORDS

So far, you have visited a patient and practiced collecting data. Now you will examine the types of available patient records and learn how to access them. The records on the Pediatric Floor and in the Surgery Department include the patient Charts, Medication Administration Record (MAR), Kardex plan of care, and Electronic Patient Record (EPR). In the Well-Child Clinic, patient records are recorded only in patient charts.

You are still signed in for Maria Ortiz on the Pediatric Floor, so let's explore her records. From the Nurses' Station, each type of patient record can be accessed in two ways. Practice both methods and choose the pathway you prefer. The first option is to use the menu in the upper left corner of the screen. First, click on **Patient Records**; this reveals a drop-down menu. Then select the type of patient record you wish to review by clicking on one of these options:

- **EPR**—Electronic Patient Record
- **Chart**—The patient's chart
- **Kardex**—A Kardex plan of care
- **MAR**—The current Medication Administration Record

You can also access patient records by clicking on various objects in the Nurses' Station. On the counter inside the station you will find a set of charts, a set of Kardex plans of care, a Medication Administration Record notebook, and a computer that houses the Electronic Patient Record system. All objects inside the Nurses' Station are labeled for quick recognition.

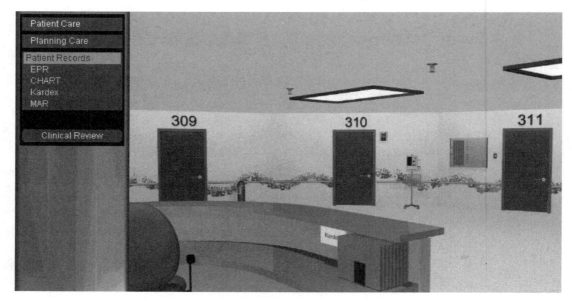

1. Chart

To open Maria's chart, click on **Chart** in the **Patient Records** drop-down menu—or click on the stack of charts inside the Nurses' Station. Colored tabs at the bottom of the screen allow you to navigate through the following sections of the chart:

- History & Physical
- Nursing History
- Admissions Records
- Physician Orders
- Progress Notes
- Laboratory Reports
- X-Rays & Diagnostics
- Operative Reports
- Medication Records
- Consults
- Rehabilitation & Therapy
- Social Services
- Miscellaneous

To flip forward in the chart, select any available tab. Once you have moved beyond the first tab (History & Physical), a **Flip Back** icon appears just above the red cross in the lower right corner. Click on **Flip Back** to return to earlier sections of the chart. The data for each patient's chart are updated during a shift; updates occur at the start of a period of care. Note that some of the records in the chart are several pages long. You will need to scroll down to read all of the pages in some sections of the chart.

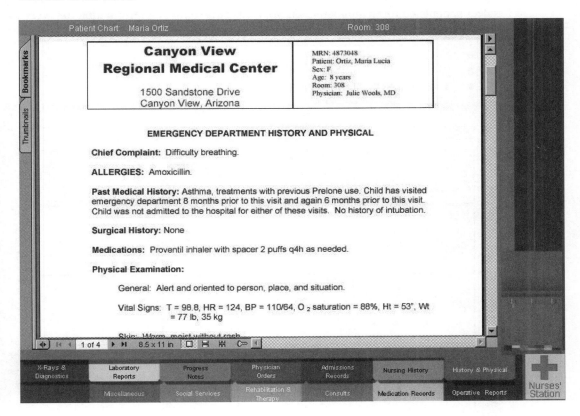

On the Pediatric Floor and in the Surgery Department, these same tabs appear in each patient's chart (see above). However, patient charts in the Well-Child Clinic have the following tabs:

- Admissions Form
- Birth & Health History
- Allergies
- Immunization Record
- Well-Child Visits
- Sick-Child Visits
- Developmental Surveillance
- Growth Charts
- Hearing & Vision Screening
- Laboratory Reports
- Referral Forms
- Anticipatory Guidance

Although the tabs differ, you navigate through the charts in the Well-Child Clinic the same way you do on the Pediatric Floor and in the Surgery Department. Flipping forward and back through the various sections is accomplished by clicking on the tabs or on the **Flip Back** icon. To close a patient's chart, click on the **Nurses' Station** icon in the lower right corner of the screen.

2. Medication Administration Record (MAR)

The notebook under the MAR sign in the Nurses' Station contains the active Medication Administration Record for each patient. This record lists the current 24-hour medications for each patient. Double-click on the MAR to open it like a notebook. (*Remember:* You can also access the MAR through the Patient Records menu.) Once open, the MAR has tabs that allow you to select patients by room number. Each MAR lists the following information for every medication a patient is receiving:

- Medication name
- Route and dosage of medication
- Time to administer medication

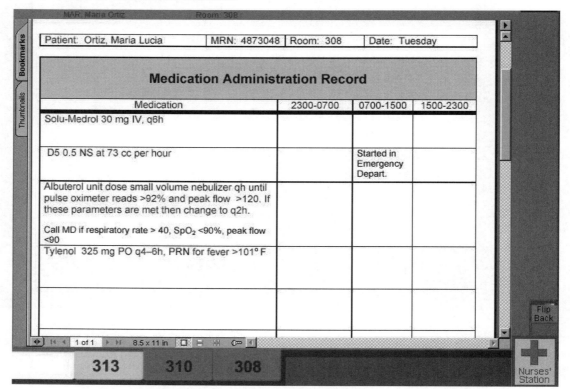

Scroll down to be sure you have read all the data. As with the patient charts, flip forward and back through the MAR by clicking on the patient room tabs or on the **Flip Back** icon. The MAR is updated at the start of every period of care. There is an MAR on the Pediatric Floor and in the Surgery Department, but not in the Well-Child Clinic. To close the MAR, click on the **Nurses' Station** icon in the lower right corner of the screen.

3. Kardex Plan of Care

Most hospitals keep a notebook in the Nurses' Station with each patient's plan of care. Canyon View Regional Medical Center's simplified plan of care is a three-page document modeled after the Kardex forms often used in hospitals. Access the Kardex through the drop-down menu (click **Patient Records**, then **Kardex**), or click on the folders beneath the Kardex sign in the Nurses' Station. Side tabs allow you to select each patient's care plan by room number. You may need to scroll down to read all of the pages.

A Flip Back icon appears in the upper right corner once you have moved past the first patient's Kardex. Use the Nurses' Station icon in the bottom right corner to return to close the Kardex.

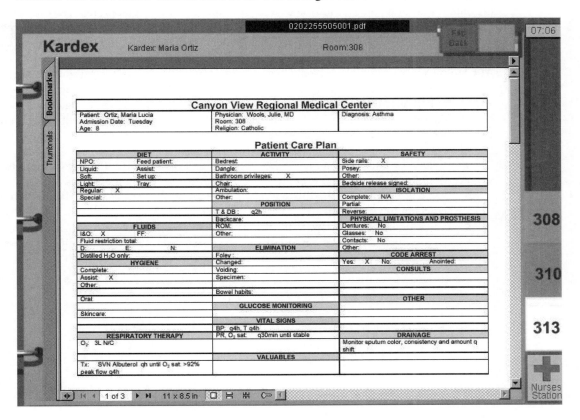

Remember: There is a Kardex on the Pediatric Floor and in the Surgery Department, but not in the Well-Child Clinic.

4. Electronic Patient Record (EPR)

Some patient records are kept in a computerized system called the Electronic Patient Record (EPR). Although some hospitals have only limited electronic patient records—or none at all—most hospitals are moving toward computerized or electronic patient record systems.

The Canyon View EPR was designed to represent a composite of commercial versions used in existing hospitals and clinics. If you have already used an EPR in a hospital, you will recognize the basic features of all commercial or custom-designed EPRs. If you have not used an EPR, the Canyon View system will give you an introduction to a very basic computerized record system.

You can use the EPR to review data already recorded for a patient—or to enter assessment data that you have collected. The EPR is continuously updated. For example, when you begin working with a patient for the 1100–1229 period of care, you have access to all the data for that patient up to 1100. The EPR contains all data collected on the patient from the moment he or she entered the hospital. The Canyon View EPR allows you to examine how data for different attributes have changed during the time the patient has been in the hospital. You may also examine data for all of a patient's attributes at a particular time. Remember, the Canyon View EPR is fully functional, as in a real hospital. Just as in real life, you can enter data during the period of care in which you are working, but you cannot change data from a previous period of care.

At Canyon View Regional Medical Center, there is an EPR system for patients on the Pediatric Floor and in the Surgery Department. The Well-Child Clinic does not have an EPR. You can access the Pediatric or Surgery EPR once you have signed in for a patient on one of those floors. Use the Patient Records menu or find the computer in the Nurses' Station with **Electronic Patient Records** on the screen. To access a patient's EPR:

- Select the EPR option on the drop-down menu (click **Patient Records**, then **EPR**) or double-click on the EPR computer screen. This will open the access screen.
- Type in the password—this will always be **nurse2b**—but **Do Not Hit Return** after entering the password.
- Click on the **Access Records** button.
- If you make a mistake, simply delete the password, reenter it, and click **Access Records**.

At the bottom of the EPR screen, you will see buttons for various types of patient data. Clicking on a button will bring up a field of attributes and the data for those attributes. You may notice that the data for some attributes appear as codes. The appropriate codes (and interpretations) for any attributes can be found in the code box on the far right side of the screen. Remember that every hospital or clinic selects its own codes. The codes used by Canyon View Regional Medical Center may be different from ones you have used or seen in clinical rotations. However, you will have to adjust to the various codes used by the clinical settings in which you work, so *Virtual Clinical Excursions—Pediatrics* gives you some practice using a system different from one you may already know. The different data fields available in the EPR are:

- Vital Signs
- Neurologic
- Musculoskeletal
- Respiratory
- Cardiovascular
- GI & GU
- IV
- Equipment
- Drains & Tubes
- Wounds & Dressings
- Hygiene
- Safety & Comfort
- Behavior & Activity
- Intake & Output

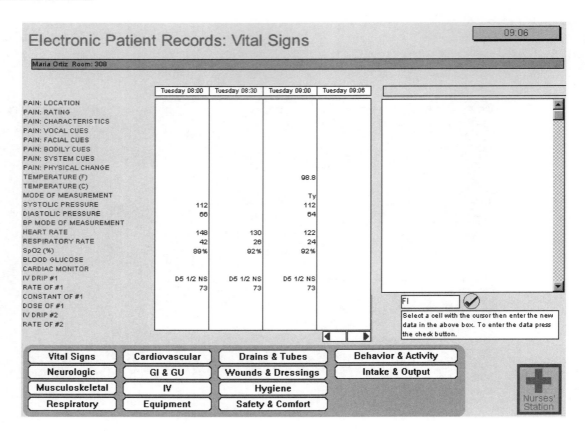

Click on **Vital Signs** and review the vital signs data for Maria Ortiz. If you want to enter data you have collected for a particular attribute (such as pain characteristics), click on the data field in which the attribute is found. (Pain characteristics are found in the Vital Signs field.) Then click on the specific attribute line, and move the highlighted box to the current time cell. Blue arrows in the lower right corner move you left and right within the EPR data fields. Once the highlighted box is in the correct time cell, type in the code for your patient's pain characteristics in the box at the lower right side of the screen, just to the left of the checkmark (√). Be sure to use the codes listed in the code box above. Once you have typed the data in this box, click on the checkmark (√) to enter them into the patient's record. The data will appear in the time cell for the attribute you have selected.

When you are ready to leave the EPR, click on the **Nurses' Station** icon in the bottom right corner of the screen.

■ PLANNING CARE

After assessing your patient, you must begin the careful process of deciding what diagnoses best describe his or her condition. For each diagnosis, you will list outcomes that you want your patient to achieve. Then, based on each outcome, you will select nursing interventions that you believe will help your patient achieve the outcomes you selected. *Virtual Clinical Excursions—Pediatrics* helps you in this process by providing a set of Planning Care resources. While you are still signed in for Maria Ortiz, click on **Planning Care** in the upper left corner of the Nurses' Station screen. You will see two options: **Problem Identification** and **Setting Priorities**.

◆ Developing Nursing Diagnoses

Click on **Problem Identification** and a note from your preceptor appears offering guidance about Maria's problems and possible diagnoses for the types of problems she may have. This diagnosis list is based on what expert nurses believe are *possible* for this particular patient. Remember, however, that not all of the diagnoses listed may apply to your patient—and that your patient may have other diagnoses that are not on the list. Your challenge and responsibility is to decide what nursing diagnoses *do* apply to your patient during each period of care. Since your patient's condition may be changing, some diagnoses may apply in one period of care but not in another. Read over the list of possible diagnoses for Maria Ortiz. When you are finished, click on **Nurses' Station** to close the Problem Identification note.

Click again on **Planning Care**. This time select **Setting Priorities**. This will open another note from your preceptor. Notice that in the third paragraph of the note, your preceptor instructs you to use the Nursing Care Matrix. This is a resource designed to help you develop nursing diagnoses for your patient. Click on **Nursing Care Matrix** at the bottom of the screen to see how. Before you can develop nursing diagnoses, you must be sure your patient actually has the characteristics of those diagnoses. It is nearly impossible for anyone to remember all of the defining characteristics for every diagnosis, so nurses consult references such as *Nursing Diagnoses: Definitions and Classification, 2001–2002* (NANDA, 2001). To make your life a little simpler and to provide training in the health informatics resources of the future, the Nursing Care Matrix provides a list of diagnoses common for your type of patient, as well as the definition for each diagnosis and the defining characteristics for each diagnosis. Ackley and Ladwig (*Nursing Diagnosis Handbook: A Guide to Planning Care*, 5th edition) have mapped specific NANDA diagnoses onto major health-illness transitions. This mapping, along with input from our expert panel of nurses, provided the list of diagnoses you see—nursing diagnoses that *might* apply to Maria Ortiz.

- Click on the first diagnosis. Note that the definition for this diagnosis now appears in a box in the upper right of the screen. The defining characteristics are listed in the box in the lower right of the screen.
- Click on another diagnosis. Review the definition and characteristics.

◆ Developing Outcomes and Interventions

For every nursing diagnosis you make, you can then select appropriate outcomes that you want your patient to achieve.

- Click on a diagnosis.
- Click on **Outcomes and Interventions** at the bottom of the screen.
- On the left-hand side of the screen, you should now see the diagnosis you selected, along with a list of the outcomes you will want your patient to achieve if she has this diagnosis.

These outcomes are based on *Nursing Outcomes Classification*, 2nd edition (Johnson, Maas, and Moorhead, 2000). This reference provides detailed lists of linkages between the NANDA diagnoses and nursing outcomes defined in the *Nursing Outcomes Classification*.

For each outcome listed, you can access a list of nursing interventions to help your patient achieve that outcome.

- Click on the first outcome.
- On the right side of your screen, you will now see lists of intervention labels in three boxes: Major Interventions, Suggested Interventions, and Optional Interventions.

Each of the intervention labels in these boxes refers to an intervention that could be implemented to help achieve the specific outcome chosen. The *Nursing Intervention Classification* system gives a label to each intervention. Therefore, the Major, Suggested, and Optional Interventions are labels, each of which has a set of nursing activities that together comprise an intervention. If you look up a label in the *Nursing Interventions Classification*, you will see that it refers to a set of different nursing activities, some or all of which can be implemented in order to achieve the desired patient outcome for that diagnosis. We used *Nursing Diagnoses, Outcomes, and Interventions: NANDA, NOC and NIC Linkages* (Johnson, Bulechek, McCloskey-Dochterman, Mass, and Moorhead, 2001) and the *Nursing Interventions Classification*, 3rd edition (McCloskey and Bulechek, 2000), to create the linkages between outcomes and interventions shown in the Nursing Care Matrix.

The Nursing Care Matrix provides you with a basic framework for learning how to move from making a diagnosis to defining patient outcomes and then to choosing the interventions you should implement to achieve those outcomes. Your instructor and the exercises in this workbook will help you develop this part of the nursing process and will provide you with more information about the nursing activities that belong with each intervention label.

■ CLINICAL REVIEW

Virtual Clinical Excursions—Pediatrics also incorporates a learning assessment system called the Clinical Review, which provides quizzes that evaluate your knowledge of your patient's condition and related conditions.

- If you are still in the Nursing Care Matrix, return to the Nurses' Station by clicking first on **Return to Diagnoses** at the bottom of the Outcomes/Interventions screen and then on **Return to Nurses' Station** at the bottom of the Diagnosis screen.
- From the menu options in the upper left corner, click on **Clinical Review**.
- You will now see a warning box that asks you to confirm that you wish to continue. Click **Clinical Review Center**.

You are now looking at the opening screen for the Clinical Review Center. Since you are working on the Pediatric Floor, you have three quiz options: **Safe Practice**, **Nursing Diagnoses**, and **Clinical Judgment**. (These same three quiz options will appear when you are working in the Surgery Department. For the Well-Child Clinic simulations, however, only the Safe Practice learning assessment is available.) Do not click on the quiz buttons yet. First, read the following descriptions of the quizzes you can select:

- **Safe Practice**
  The **Safe Practice** quiz presents you with NCLEX-RN–type questions based on the patient you worked with during this period of care. A set of five questions is randomly drawn from a pool of questions. Answer the questions, and the Clinical Review Center will score your performance.

- **Nursing Diagnoses**
  If you click on the **Nursing Diagnoses** button, you are presented with a list of 20 NANDA nursing diagnoses. You must select the five diagnoses in this list that most likely apply to your patient. The Clinical Review Center records your choices, gathers those choices that are correct, and scores your performance. The quiz then allows you

to select nursing interventions for each of the outcomes associated with NANDA diagnoses that your correctly chose. For each of your correct diagnoses, you are presented with the likely outcomes for that diagnosis; for each outcome, you will see a list of six nursing intervention labels. Only three of the intervention labels are appropriate for each outcome. You must select the correct labels. Again, your performance is automatically scored.

- **Clinical Judgement**
  The **Clinical Judgment** quiz asks you to consider a single question. This question evaluates your understanding of your patient's condition during the period of care in which you have just worked. Select your answer from four options related to your perception of your patient's stability and the frequency of monitoring you should be conducting.

On the Pediatrics Floor and in the Surgery Department, you can take one, two, or all three of the quizzes. In the Well-Child Clinic, you can only take the **Safe Practice** quiz. On any floor, when you are done with the quizzes, you must click on **Finish**. This will take you to a **Preceptor's Evaluation**, which offers a scorecard of your performance on the quizzes, discusses your understanding of the patient's condition and related conditions, and makes recommendations for you to improve your understanding.

Preceptor's Evaluation

	Correct Responses	Score
Safe Practice	3.0	18.0
Implementing Nursing Care	3.0	12.0
Clinical Judgment	0	0
Totals		30.0
Total Score	Out of 100 possible points, you received 30.0 points or 30.0%	

Preceptor's Evaluation of Clinical Review

Clincial Judgment Recommendation - We do not agree with your judgment about the client's status. Please review your assessment data and reconsider your evaluation of this patient

We want you to spend time practicing questions like those found in the Safe Practice assessment. These questions are very similar to those found on the NCLEX-RN. Also, we feel you need to study the nursing diagnoses approved by the North American Nursing Diagnosis Association (NANDA). Importantly, we want you to review the outcomes appropriate for a particular diagnosis as well as the interventions you would implement to achieve each outcome. You might want to spend time re-examining the diagnoses-outcomes-interventions linkages found in the Nursing Care Matrix. As mentioned above, the nursing diagnoses are based on approved diagnoses of the North American Nursing Diagnosis Association (NANDA). Remember that the outcomes are based on the Nursing Outcomes Classification and the interventions are based on the Nursing Interventions Classification (NIC).

Print Detailed Report   Nurses' Station

Note: We don't recommend that you take any quizzes before working with a patient. The goal of *Virtual Clinical Excursions—Pediatrics* is to help you learn and prepare for practice as a professional nurse. Reading your textbook, using this workbook to complete the CD-ROM activities, and organizing your thoughts about your patient's condition will help you prepare for the quizzes. More important, this work will help you prepare for care of real-life patients in clinical settings.

■ HOW TO QUIT OR CHANGE PATIENTS

Eventually, you will want to take a short or long break, begin caring for a different patient, or exit the software.

◆ To Take a Short Break

- Go to the Nurses' Station.
- Click on **Leave the Floor**, an icon in the lower left corner of the screen.
- You will see a screen with a variety of options.
- Click on **Break** and you will be given a 10-minute break. This stops the clock. After 10 minutes you are automatically returned to the floor, where you reenter the simulation at the same moment in time that you left.

◆ To Change Patients

Choose option 1 or option 2 below, depending on which activities you have completed during this period of care.

1. Use the following instructions *if you have already completed one or more of the quizzes* in the Clinical Review Center for your current patient:

   - Double-click on the Supervisor's (Login) Computer in the Nurses' Station.
   - Read the instructions for logging in for a new patient and period of care.
   - If you want to select a new patient on the *same* floor, click **Login**, select the new patient and period of care, and then click **Nurses' Station**.
   - If you want to work with a patient on a *different* floor, click **Return to Nurses' Station**, take the elevator to that floor, and sign in for the new patient on the Login computer in the Nurses' Station.

2. Use the following instructions *if you have* not *completed any of the quizzes* in the Clinical Review Center for your current patient:

   - Double-click on the Supervisor's (Login) Computer in the Nurses' Station.
   - Read the instructions in the Warning box. Then click on **Supervisor's Computer**.
   - The computer logs you off and gives you the option of going to the Clinical Review Center or to the Nurses' Station. Unless you wish to go to the Clinical Review Center for evaluation of the period of care you just completed, click on **Nurses' Station**.
   - Double-click on the Login Computer again, and follow the instructions to sign in for another patient. (See the third and fourth bullets in option 1 above for specific steps.)

◆ **To Quit the Software for a Long Break or to Reset a Simulation**

- From the Nurses' Station, click on **Leave the Floor** in the lower left corner of the screen.
- You will see a new screen with a variety of options.
- You may select Quit with Bookmark or Quit with Reset.
  - **Quit with Bookmark** allows you to leave the simulation and return at the same virtual time you left. Any data you entered in the EPR will remain intact. Choose this option if you want to stop working for more than 10 minutes but wish to reenter the floor later at the exact point at which you left.
  - **Quit with Reset** allows you to quit and reset the simulation. This option erases any data you entered in the EPR during your current session. Choose this option if you know you will be starting a new simulation when you return.

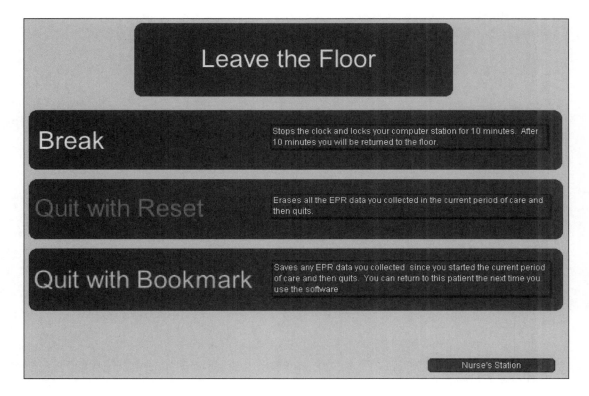

◆ **To Practice Exiting the Software**

- Click **Leave the Floor**.
- Now click **Quit with Reset**.
- A small message box will appear to confirm that you wish to quit and erase any data collected or recorded.
  - If you have reached this message in error, click the red X in the upper right corner to close this box. You may now choose one of the other options for leaving the floor (Break or Quit with Bookmark).
  - If you *do* wish to Quit with Reset, click **OK** on the message box.
- *Virtual Clinical Excursions—Pediatrics* will close and you will be returned to your computer's desktop screen.

A DETAILED TOUR

What do you experience when you care for patients during a clinical rotation? Well, you may be assigned one or several patients that need your attention. You follow the nursing process, assessing your patients, diagnosing each patient's problems or areas of concern, planning their care and setting outcomes you hope they will achieve, implementing care based on the outcomes you have set, and then evaluating the outcomes of your care. It is so important to remember that the nursing process is not a static, one-time series of steps. Instead, you loop through the process again and again, continuously assessing your patient, reaffirming your earlier diagnoses and perhaps finding improvement in some areas and new problems in other areas, adjusting your plan of care, implementing care as planned or implementing a revised plan, and evaluating patient outcomes to decide whether your patients are achieving expected outcomes. Patient care is hands-on, action-packed, often complex, and sometimes frightening. You must be prepared and present—physically, intellectually, and emotionally.

Textbooks help you build a foundation of knowledge about patient care. Clinical rotations help you apply and extend that book-based learning to the real world. You will know this with certainty when you experience it yourself—for example, when you first read about starting an IV but then have to start an IV on an actual patient, or when you read about the adverse effects of a medication and you then observe these adverse effects emerging in a patient. Stepping from a book onto a hospital floor seems difficult and unsettling. *Virtual Clinical Excursions—Pediatrics* is designed to help you make the transition from book-based learning to the real world of patient care. The CD-ROM activities provide you with the practice necessary to make that transition by letting you apply your book-based knowledge to virtual patients in simulated settings and situations. Each simulation was developed by an expert nurse or nurse-physician team and is based on realistic patient problems, with a rich variety of data that can be collected during assessment of the patient.

Several types of patient records are available for you to access and analyze. This workbook, the software, and your textbook work together to allow you to move from ***book-based learning*** to real-life ***problem-based learning***. Your foundational knowledge is based on what you have learned from the textbook. The *VCE—Pediatrics* patient simulations allow you to explore this knowledge in the context of a virtual hospital with virtual patients. Questions stimulated by the software can be answered by consulting your textbook or reviewing a patient simulation. The workbook is similar to a map or guide, providing a means of connecting textbook content to the practice of skills, data collection, and data interpretation by leading you through a variety of relevant activities based on simulated patients' conditions.

To better understand how *Virtual Clinical Excursions—Pediatrics* can help you in your transition, take the following detailed tour, in which you visit three different patients.

■ WORKING WITH A PEDIATRIC FLOOR PATIENT

In *Virtual Clinical Excursions—Pediatrics*, the Pediatric Floor can be visited between 0700 and 1500, but you can care for only one patient at a time and only in the following blocks of time, which we call *periods of care*: 0700–0829, 0900–1029, 1100–1229, and 1300–1429. For each clinical simulation, you will select a single patient and a period of care. When you have completed the assigned care for that patient, you can then select a new patient and period of care. You can also reset a simulation at any point and work through the same period of care as many times as you want. Each time you sign in for a patient and time period, you will enter that session at the beginning of that period of care (unless you have previously "saved" a session by choosing Break or Quit with Bookmark).

Consider, for a moment, a typical Pediatric Floor during the period between 0700 and 1500. Suppose that you could accompany a preceptor on that floor and provide care for patients during that 8-hour shift. Different expert nurses might take slightly different approaches, but almost certainly each nurse would establish priorities for patient care. These priorities would be based on report during shift change, a review of the patient records, and the nurse's own assessment of each patient.

At the beginning of a period of care, the assessment of each patient is usually accomplished by a general survey, that is, a fairly complete assessment of a patient's physical and psychosocial status. After the general survey, a nurse subsequently conducts focused assessments during the rest of the shift. The specific types of data collected in such focused assessments are determined by the nurse's interpretation of each patient's condition, needs, and applicable clinical pathways for independent and collaborative care. Depending on an agency's protocols and standards of care for the pediatric patient, a nurse may conduct more than one comprehensive assessment during a shift, with focused surveys completed between the general surveys. Regardless of individual agency protocol, any pediatric floor patient would have at least one general survey and two or more focused surveys over the period of the shift.

Now let's put these guidelines to practice by returning to the Pediatric Floor at Canyon View Regional Medical Center. This time, you will care for De Olp, a 6-year-old girl with leukemia.

1. Enter and Sign In for De Olp

- Insert your *VCE—Pediatrics* **Patients' Disk** in your CD-ROM drive and double-click on the **VCE—Pediatrics** icon on your desktop. Wait for the program to load.
- When Canyon View Regional Medical Center appears on your screen, click on the hospital entrance to enter the lobby.
- Click on the elevator. Once inside, click on the panel to the right of the door; then click on button **3** for the Pediatric Floor.
- When the elevator opens onto the Pediatric Floor, click on the **Nurses' Station**.
- Inside the Nurses' Station, double-click on the **Supervisor's (Login) Computer** and select De Olp as your patient for the 0900–1029 period of care.

2. Case Overview

- Signing in automatically takes you to the patient's Case Overview. Your preceptor will appear and speak briefly on the video screen.
- Listen to the preceptor; then click on **Assignment** below the video screen.
- You will now see a Preceptor Note, which is a summary of care for De Olp, covering the period of care just before the one you are now working.
- Review the summary of care. Scroll down to read the entire report.
- On the next page, make note of any information that you feel is important or that will require follow-up work, either with the patient or through examination of her records.

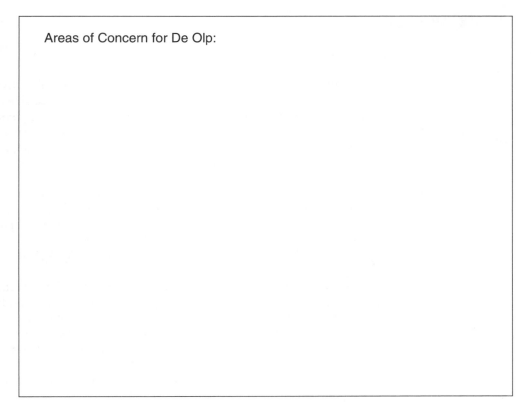

Areas of Concern for De Olp:

- When you have finished the case overview, click on **Nurses' Station** in the lower right corner of the screen and you will find yourself in the Pediatric Nurses' Station.

3. Initial Impressions

Visit your patient immediately to get an initial impression of her condition.

- On the menu in the upper left corner of your screen, click on **Patient Care**. From the options on the drop-down menu, click on **Data Collection**. *Remember:* You can also visit the patient by double-clicking on the door to her room (Room 310).
- In the anteroom, wash your hands by double-clicking on the sink. Then click on the curtain to enter the patient area.
- Inside the room, you will see many different options for assessing this patient. First, click on **Initial Observations** in the top left corner of the screen. Observe and listen to the interaction between the nurse preceptor and the patient. Note any areas of concern, issues, or assessments that you may want to pursue later.
- Now that you have gotten an initial impression of you patient, you have a few choices. In some cases, you might wish to leave the patient and access her records to develop a better understanding of her condition and what has happened since she was admitted. However, let's stay with De a while longer to conduct a few physical and psychosocial assessments.

4. Vital Signs

Obtain a full set of vital signs from De Olp.

- Click on **Vital Signs** (just below the Initial Observations button). This activates a pathway that allows you to measure all or just some of your patient's vital signs. Four options now appear under the picture of De Olp. Clicking on any of these options will begin a data collection sequence (usually a short video) in which the respective vital sign is measured. The vital signs data change over time to reflect the temporal changes you would find in a patient such as De. Try the various vital signs options to see what kinds of data are obtained.
  - First, click on **BP/SpO$_2$/HR**. Wait for the video to begin; then observe as the nurse preceptor uses a noninvasive monitor to measure De's blood pressure, SpO$_2$, and heart rate. After the video stops, the preceptor's findings appear as digital readings on a monitor to the right of the video screen. Record these data in the chart below. If you want to replay the video, simply click again on **BP/SpO$_2$/HR**. *Note:* You can replay any video in this manner—as often as needed.
  - Now click on **Respiratory Rate**. This time, after the video plays, an image of a breathing body model appears on the right. Count the respirations for the amount of time recommended by your instructor. Record your measurement below.
  - Next, click on **Temperature**. Again, a video shows the nurse preceptor obtaining this vital sign, and the result is shown on a close-up of a digital thermometer on the right side of the screen. Record this finding in the chart below.
  - Finally, click on **Pain Assessment** and observe as the nurse preceptor asks De about her pain. Note De's response in the chart below.

Vital Signs	Time
Blood pressure	
SpO$_2$	
Heart rate	
Respiratory rate	
Temperature	
Pain rating	

5. Mental Status

From some of your vital signs assessments, you should be starting to form an idea of De's mental status. However, you can check her mental status more specifically by doing the following:

- On the left side of the Data Collection screen is a body model. When you move your cursor along the body, it begins to rotate and the area beneath your cursor is highlighted in orange.
- Place your cursor on the head area of the body model and click.
- Notice that new assessment options now appear under the picture of your patient.
- Click on **Mental Status** (the bottom option of the list).
- Observe De's responses and interactions with the nurse. Then review the data, if any, that appear to the right after the video has stopped.

6. Respiratory Assessment

De Olp has received medication that may cause fluid retention. Auscultate her lungs to see whether there is any evidence of edema.

- Click on the chest area of the body model.
- Note the new assessment options that come up beneath the picture of De.
- Click on **Respiratory**.
- Observe the examination of the anterior, lateral, and posterior chest. Then review the data collected by your preceptor.
- Do you believe there is any evidence of pulmonary edema? If so, explain what data support your conclusion.
- If you were worried about fluid retention, what other assessments might you conduct?

7. Behavior

Since this is your first visit with De, you may also want to collect some psychosocial data.

- At the bottom left corner of the screen, click on **Behavior**.
- One at a time, click on each of the behavioral assessment options that appear below the picture of De.
- As you observe each assessment, take notes on the nurse-patient interactions.
- Do any of De's responses concern you?
- Does De have family support as well as nursing support?
- What other questions do you want to ask De? When might you ask these questions?

8. Chart

You have conducted your preliminary examination of De. Next, review her patient records.

- To access the patient charts, either click on the stack of charts inside the Nurses' Station or click on **Patient Records** and then **Chart** from the drop-down menu.
- De Olp's chart automatically appears since you are signed in to care for her. As described earlier in **A Quick Tour**, the chart is divided into several sections. Each section is marked by a colored tab at the bottom of the screen. To flip forward and back through the chart sections, click on the labeled tabs and on the **Flip Back** icon, respectively. Once you have moved beyond a section, the tab for that section disappears. You can move back to previous sections *only* by clicking on the **Flip Back** icon, which appears above the Nurses' Station icon in the lower right corner.
- Review the following sections of De's chart: History & Physical, Nursing History, Operative Reports, and Progress Notes.

- Based on your analyses of these records and your preliminary assessment of De, summarize key issues for this patient's care in the box below.
- When you are finished, close the chart by clicking on the **Nurses' Station** icon.

Key Issues for Patient Care:

---

9. Electronic Patient Record (EPR)

Now examine the data in De Olp's EPR.

- To access the EPR, first click **Patient Records** in the upper left corner of the screen. Then click **EPR** on the drop-down menu. *Remember:* As an alternative, you can also double-click on the EPR computer in the Nurses' Station. This computer is located to the left of the Kardex and has **Electronic Patient Records** on the screen.
- On the access screen, enter the password—**nurse2b**—and click **Access Records**.
- The EPR automatically opens to the patient's Vital Signs summary. Examine De Olp's vital signs data for the past 8 hours.
- Now click **Respiratory** (three buttons below Vital Signs). The data from assessments of De's respiratory system are now shown.
- De has been receiving a medication that may cause some fluid retention. Review the data for her lung auscultation to determine where there is any evidence of pulmonary edema. Record your findings in the box on the next page.

Lung Sounds During the Past 24 Hours:

- Click on **Cardiovascular**.
- Review data collected for edema.
- List any evidence for fluid retention as evidenced by edema.
- Make sure that if edema was observed, you note the locations and quality.
- Now, make an assessment of De's clinical status:

  a. Are any of the vital signs data you collected this morning significantly different from the baselines for those vital signs?

      Circle One: Yes   No

  b. If "Yes," which data are different?

  c. Do you have any concerns about the data collected during your respiratory assessment?

      Circle One: Yes   No

  d. If you answered "No," what data tell you the patient is stable?

  e. If you answered "Yes," what are your concerns?

10. Medication Administration Record (MAR)

- De has been taking a number of medications. Access her current MAR by double-clicking on the notebook below the MAR sign in the Nurse' Station. You can also open the MAR by clicking on **Patient Records** and then on **MAR** on the drop-down menu.
- Once the MAR notebook is open, access De's records by clicking on the tab with her room number (310) at the bottom of the screen.
- Examine the MAR and note any medications that De should be given during the period of care between 0900 and 1029. Make a list of these medications, the times they are to be administered, and any assessments you should conduct before and after giving the medications.
- Click the **Nurses' Station** icon to close the MAR.

11. Planning Care

So far, you have completed a preliminary examination of De Olp and reviewed some of her records. Now you can begin to plan her care. *Note:* Before *actually* starting a plan of care, you would conduct a more thorough assessment and a more complete review of this patient's records. However, let's continue so that you can learn how to use *Virtual Clinical Excursion's* unique and valuable Planning Care resource.

- On the drop-down menu, click **Planning Care** and then **Problem Identification**.
- Read the Preceptor Note on problem identification for De Olp and write one nursing diagnosis that you think might apply to this patient. Base you decision on your preliminary assessment and review of her records.
- Click on **Nurses' Station** to close this note.
- Click again on **Planning Care** in the upper left corner of your screen. This time, select **Setting Priorities** from the drop-down menu.
- Review the Preceptor Note on setting priorities for De.
- When you have finished, click on **Nursing Care Matrix** at the bottom of your screen.
- You will now see a list of nursing diagnoses approved by the North American Nursing Diagnosis Association (NANDA) that may apply to De's condition.
- Find the diagnosis you just identified for De. Click on this diagnosis.
- Review the nursing diagnosis definition and the defining characteristics that now appear on the right side of the screen.
- Does the definition fit your patient?
- Does your patient have the defining characteristics? If not, perhaps your assessment was not complete enough for you to make this decision. What other assessments should you conduct in order to determine whether this diagnosis applies to De Olp?
- For now, assume that your diagnosis *does* apply to De. Click on the **Outcomes and Interventions** button at the bottom of the screen.
- You now see a screen that lists nursing outcomes for your diagnosis. These are based on the Nursing Outcomes Classification. If your patient has this diagnosis, these are the outcomes you will want her to achieve.
- Some or all of these outcomes will probably apply to your patient if she does indeed have the nursing diagnosis you selected.
- Click on the first outcome, and text will appear in the three boxes on the right side of the screen. These boxes show the Major, Suggested, and Optional Interventions that could be implemented to achieve the outcome you selected, based on the Nursing Interventions Classification. *Remember:* Each entry listed in these boxes is an intervention label that represents a *set* of nursing activities that you would implement.
- Review the nursing interventions, especially those in the Major Interventions box. These are the most likely interventions you would implement to achieve the outcome you have clicked. However, you should consider all of the interventions before deciding which apply to the outcome for your patient.

- Now click on **Return to Diagnoses**. At this time, you can explore other diagnoses and their respective outcomes and interventions, or you can click **Return to Nurses' Station**.

Your work with De Olp is completed for now. To quit the software and reset a simulation:

- Go to the Nurses' Station.
- Click on **Leave the Floor** in the lower left corner of the screen.
- A screen appears with a variety of options.
- Select **Quit with Reset**, which allows you to quit and reset the simulation. This option erases any data you entered in the EPR during your current session.

■ WORKING WITH A WELL-CHILD CLINIC PATIENT

In *Virtual Clinical Excursions—Pediatrics*, the Well-Child Clinic can be visited between 0700 and 1100. You can visit three different patients, but you can visit only one child at a time. Entering the clinic and selecting a patient begins a Well-Child Clinic visit in which you work with two professional nurses, one of whom is a pediatric nurse practitioner. This time, you will care for 24-month-old Paul Parker, who is accompanied by his mother.

1. Enter and Sign In for Paul Parker

- Insert your *VCE—Pediatrics* **Patients' Disk** in your CD-ROM drive and double-click on the **VCE—Pediatrics** icon on your desktop. Wait for the program to load.
- When Canyon View Regional Medical Center appears on your screen, click on the hospital entrance to enter the lobby.
- Click on the elevator. Once inside, click on the panel to the right of the door; then click on **2** for the Well-Child Clinic.
- When the elevator arrives at the Well-Child Clinic, click on the **Nurses' Station** to enter the clinic.
- You will use only one computer at this Nurses' Station—the Supervisor's (Login) Computer. Find this computer and double-click on the screen.
- Click **Login**.

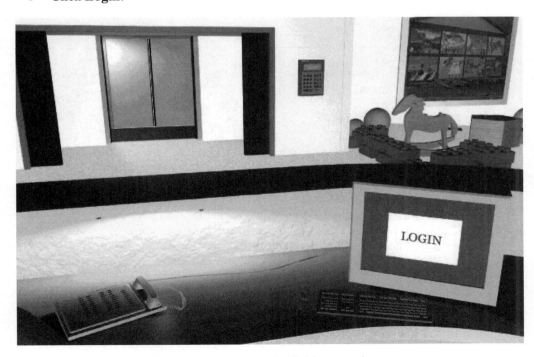

- Select Paul Parker as your patient. (*Note*: Only one period of care is available.)
- Click **Nurses' Station** in the lower right corner.

2. Case Overview

- Signing in automatically takes you to the patient's Case Overview.
- Listen to the preceptor; then click on **Assignment** below the video screen.
- Read the Preceptor Note, which summarizes important information about conducting a well-child visit and assigns specific tasks for you to complete during the visit.
- Below, note any information that you feel is important to remember when you examine a pediatric patient during a well-child visit.

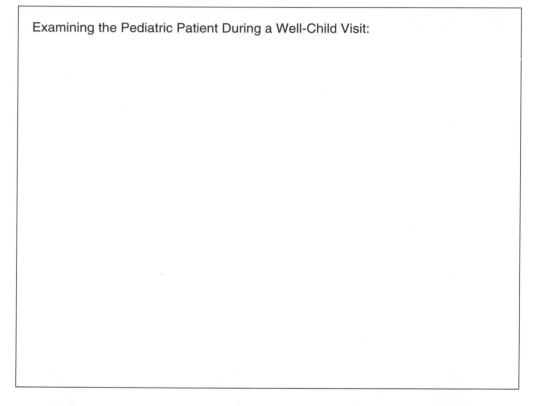

Examining the Pediatric Patient During a Well-Child Visit:

- Click on **Nurses' Station** to complete the Case Overview and return to the Well-Child Clinic Nurses' Station.

3. Preliminary Examination

Visit your patient immediately to complete a preliminary examination.

- Review the menu of options in the upper left corner of your screen.
- Click on **Physical Examination**.
- In the anteroom, double-click on the sink to wash your hands. Then click on the curtain to the right of the sink and enter the examination room.
- Click on **Preliminary Examination** at the upper left side of the screen. Notice that a list of additional assessment options for this selection appears under the picture of your patient.
- Experiment by clicking the options one at a time. After clicking each option, wait for the video to begin; then follow the professional nurse through each portion of the preliminary examination of Paul Parker.

- As you observe the assessments, make note of the types of data that are collected.
- You probably noticed that for some of the assessment options, the video does not show all of the assessments for which data appeared to the right of the video screen. Form a small collaborative group with a few of your classmates. Discuss which assessments were incomplete or missing during the preliminary examination. Identify the specific type of assessment that would yield each of the results shown to the right of the video screen. Take turns critiquing the techniques used by the nurse in the videos. Discuss what you might do differently.

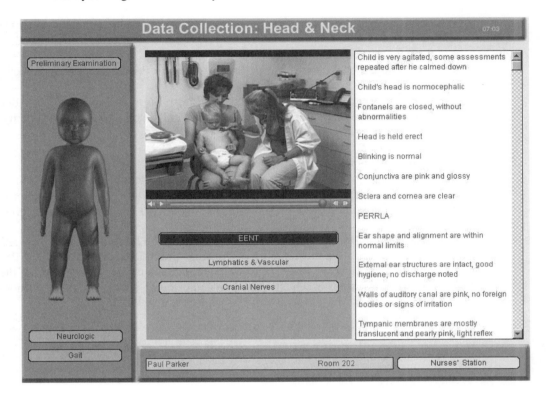

4. Other Well-Child Assessments

Now that you have observed Paul Parker's preliminary examination, conduct a physical examination of this patient by clicking on various parts of the body model. This time, you will work with the nurse practitioner. *Note:* If you receive a message telling you that the current period of care has ended (or if the clock on your screen shows that time for this visit has almost expired), go back to the Supervisor's (Login) Computer and log in for Paul Parker a second time. Simply double-click on the Login screen and follow instructions for selecting another patient—but reselect Paul Parker instead.

- First, click on the head area of the body model.
- The following assessment options appear for the head and neck area of the patient: EENT, Lymphatics & Vascular, and Cranial Nerves.
- Click on each of the options, watching the videos and examining the findings of the nurse practitioner. Describe some of the problems the nurse practitioner encounters, for example, when she tries to examine Paul's nose, mouth, and ears. Is there anything she could do differently in order to help Paul feel comfortable with an ear examination?
- Now click on the chest area of the body model.
- What types of assessment options are available?
- Watch these assessments, analyzing the data obtained from each assessment.

- Decide whether the data collected indicate any problems with Paul's respiratory or cardiovascular system. If you determined there were some problem areas, what other assessments would you want to do? What other data would you want to collect to investigate these problems in more detail?

5. Parent Interview

Now take some time to visit with Paul's mother.

- From the examination room, return to the Nurses' Station. Which button do you click to get there?
- *Remember*: You must stop to wash your hands in the anteroom.
- Once you are back in the Nurses' Station, click on **Parent Interview** (upper left side of the screen).
- On the Parent Interview screen, click on **Health Supervision** below the video monitor.
- Observe the nurse practitioner interviewing Paul's mother. Take notes on any important issues raised during these discussions.
- Now click on **Developmental Observations**.
- Again, take notes on the nurse-parent discussions.
- Based on the parent interview, how would you decide whether Paul's mother provides a safe environment for her child and follows good health supervision practices?
- How would you decide whether Paul is at the developmental stage appropriate for his age?
- Return to the Nurses' Station. This time click on the **Developmental Surveillance** button. This accesses a summary of the nurse practitioner's assessment of Paul's developmental status. Based on your examination and your observation of the parent interview, list areas in which you agree and disagree with the nurse practitioner. For example, does Paul's mother say that he does not attend day care?

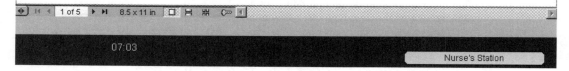

Developmental Assessment Summary of Findings

Patient name: Paul Parker

Age at testing: 2 years

Date of birth: 4/15

Findings: Paul was tested in four categories today for developmental progress. These categories were motor skills, language skills, social skills and cognitive ability. In the language and cognitive skills assessment, Paul was found to be speaking frequently, but most of his words sound the same. Some phrases are understandable, and he appears to understand what is spoken to him. He follows simple commands well. According to mom, Paul is able to obey commands at home and understands what she tells him. Paul is being referred to a speech therapist at this time for evaluation of speech development progress. In the area of motor skills, Paul is doing well. He is able to walk up stairs, kick a ball, and feed himself, and he is beginning to toilet train. Socially, Paul is a shy toddler, he does not attend day care and has a sibling, age 4, at home. He is exhibiting some aggressive and selfish behavior toward his sibling. This behavior is normal for a child of Paul's age.

Impression: Paul is on target for developmental skills in cognitive, motor, and social areas and is being referred to a specialist for language development assessment.

1 of 5   8.5 x 11 in

07:03

Nurse's Station

6. Chart

- Access Paul Parker's chart by double-clicking on the stack of charts in the Nurses' Station or by clicking **Patient Records** from the menu on the left side of the screen.
- Read the following sections of Paul's chart: Birth & Health History, Immunization Record, Well-Child Visits, Sick-Child Visits, and Growth Charts.
- Based on your analyses of these records, do you find any reasons why Paul may be sensitive about having his ears examined? List and describe other key issues for this patient's care.
- Plot Paul's length and weight on the Growth Charts. Do his measurements fall within reasonable ranges for his age?
- Are Paul's immunizations current? If not, how would you discuss with his mother the need to complete immunizations?
- Below, list any other areas that are key issues for Paul.

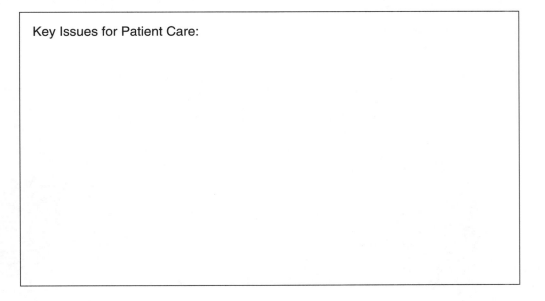

Key Issues for Patient Care:

Remember: The Well-Child Clinic does not have a Medication Administration Record, a Kardex plan of care, or an Electronic Patient Record. This clinic is an outpatient service provided by Canyon View Regional Medical Center, and although an EPR would be of value, the costs have prohibited its extension to the Well-Child Clinic. In an ideal setting, all patient records would be available in a computerized system, including data from every visit to the hospital or any of its associated outpatient clinics. Specifically, think about how such an EPR system would be useful to nurses in the Well-Child Clinic? How could an EPR provide data that are not already available in the chart?

It is time to leave the Well-Child Clinic. Before you can go to another floor, you must log out from your current patient:

- Double-click on the Supervisor's Computer.
- Read the Warning message that explains how to log off.
- Click on the **Supervisor's Computer** button.
- The next screen asks you whether you want to visit the Clinical Review Center (for evaluation of your work with Paul Parker) or return to the Nurses' Station.
- We want to work with a new patient now, so click **Nurses' Station**.
- Take the elevator to the Pediatric Floor and begin the next section, Working with a Perioperative Patient.

■ WORKING WITH A PERIOPERATIVE PATIENT

One of the pediatric patients at Canyon View Regional Medical Center, Jason Baker, has a badly fractured leg.

- On the Pediatric Floor, sign in to visit Jason for his Preoperative Interview.
- The interview takes place in Jason's room, so click on **Patient Care** and then **Data Collection** on the drop-down menu.
- Wash your hands, enter the room, and click **View Interview**.
- After observing the interview, click on **Summary** and read the Preceptor Note.
- Now return to the Nurses' Station and sign out so that you can go to the Surgery Department, where Jason has been transported for Preoperative Care.
- Take the elevator to the 4th floor. Click on the Nurses' Station and sign in to visit Jason during his preoperative care.
- Although you cannot observe Jason's surgery, you can see him now in the Preoperative Care Bay and later in the PACU
- Once Jason is transferred out of PACU, you can visit him in his room on the Pediatric Floor.

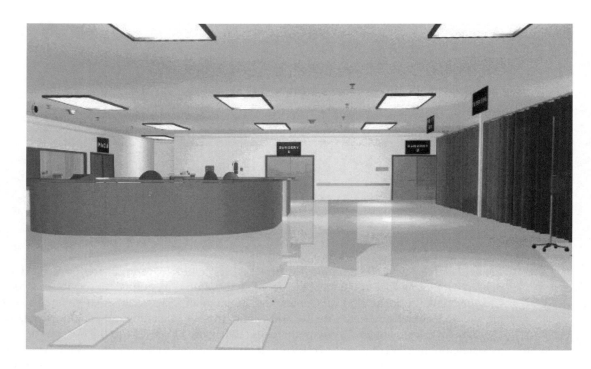

- Spend some time in each of the different perioperative settings described on p. 42. Then compare these perioperative settings with the settings on the Pediatric Floor and in the Well-Child Clinic. Use the following chart and focus your comparisons on the themes listed in the left column.

Comparison of Settings in Canyon View Regional Medical Center			
Activities and Resources	**Perioperative Settings**	**Pediatric Floor Settings**	**Well-Child Clinic Settings**
Patient Assessments			
Planning Care			
Types of Patient Records			

Remember: *Virtual Clinical Excursions—Pediatrics* is designed to provide a realistic learning environment. Within Canyon View Regional Medical Center, you will not necessarily find the same type of patient records, clinical settings, Nurses' Station layout, or hospital floor architecture that you find in your real-life clinical rotations. If you have already had experience within actual clinical settings, take a few moments to list the similarities and differences between the Canyon View virtual hospital and the real hospitals you have visited. There is considerable variation among hospitals in the United States, so think of *Virtual Clinical Excursions—Pediatrics* as simply one type of hospital and take advantage of the opportunity to practice learning how, where, when, and why to find the information, medication, and equipment resources you need to provide the highest quality patient care.

The following icons are used throughout the workbook to help you quickly identify particular activities and assignments:

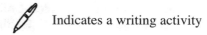 Indicates a reading assignment—tells you which textbook chapter(s) you should read before starting each lesson

Indicates a writing activity

Marks the beginning of an interactive CD-ROM activity—signals you to open or return to your *Virtual Clinical Excursions—Pediatrics* Patients' Disk

Indicates a continuation of CD-ROM instructions

Indicates questions and activities that require you to consult your textbook

LESSON **1**

Family-Centered Nursing Care

⚬⚬ **Reading Assignment:** Family-Centered Nursing Care (Chapter 2)
Nursing Care of the Child with a Psychosocial Disorder
(Chapter 30): Section on Child Abuse and Neglect

Patients: Sherrie Bedonie, 4 years old, Well-Child Clinic, Room 204
Matthew Brown, 10 months old, Well-Child Clinic, Room 205
Jason Baker, 14 years old, Pediatric Unit, Room 306
Kaylie Sern, 3 years old, Pediatric Unit, Room 304

This lesson focuses on the importance of the family both in the lives of children and in their health care. Different types of families are discussed, giving the student the opportunity to assess the families of four different children: two children in the Well-Child Clinic and two children in the Pediatric Unit. Sherrie Bedonie, age 4 years, lives in a two-parent family. Matthew Brown's mother died in an accident 2 months ago, and his father is grieving over the loss of his wife and the change in his parenting role. Kaylie Sern, age 3 years, is being cared for by foster parents. Jason Baker's parents are divorced; his mother is remarried, and his biological father lives out of state. For each of these patients, you will be given the opportunity to assess the family, draw conclusions, and recognize the stressors inherent in the family. In addition to family-centered care, this lesson addresses child abuse and neglect and their effect on children and families.

Objectives

Upon completion of this lesson, you will be able to:

1. Identify different types of families.
2. Conduct a Friedman Family Assessment of two families.
3. Write a nursing care plan to support a grieving father.
4. Construct a genogram and an ecomap of two different families.
5. Develop insight into the dysfunctional family.
6. Discuss child abuse and neglect as it relates to children and families.
7. Identify the legal requirements regarding the reporting of suspected child abuse and/or neglect.

In your textbook, read the sections on family types, family theories, and parenting in Chapter 2, pp. 29-37.

1. Using Box 2-1 (p. 34 in your textbook), describe the characteristics that make up the healthy family.

2. How do the characteristics of parents and children influence their relationship?

CD-ROM Activity

Open your *Virtual Clinical Excursions—Pediatrics* Patients' Disk. Enter the lobby of Canyon View Regional Medical Center and take the elevator to the **Well-Child Clinic (Floor 2)**. While on the floor, you will visit two well children in order to study their family structures.

From the elevator, click on the **Nurses' Station** and sign in on the **Login Computer** to see Sherrie Bedonie for her routine well-child visit at 08:30 in Room 204. After listening to the Case Overview, return to the Nurses' Station and open Sherrie's Chart by clicking on **Patient Records**. (*Remember:* You can also access her Chart by clicking on the stack of charts on the counter of the Nurses' Station.) Click on the appropriate tabs at the bottom of the Chart to open and review the following sections: **Admissions Form**, **Birth & Health History**, and **Well-Child Visits**. As you read, record any data you wish to remember under Sherrie's name below and on the next page.

Now return to the **Nurses' Station** and click on **Parent Interview**. Observe the interview with Sherrie's mother by clicking on **Health Supervision** and then on **Developmental Observations**. As you listen, record any important points below and on the next page.

Student Notes	Sherrie Bedonie	Matthew Brown
History regarding family		
Observations from visiting with the family		

	Sherrie Bedonie	Matthew Brown

Any additional
information

→ Once you have finished visiting and learning about Sherrie and her family, return to the Nurses'
Station and click on the **Login Computer**. Select the **Supervisor's Computer** icon to sign out
from caring for Sherrie. Then click on the button that says **Return to the Nurses' Station** and
once again click on the **Login Computer**, this time selecting Matthew Brown at 10:00 in Room
205. Matthew is a 10-month-old boy who has also come to the Well-Child Clinic for his routine
check-up. Just as you did with Sherrie, review his family history by clicking on **Patient
Records** and reviewing these sections of his Chart: Admissions Form, Birth & Health History,
and Well-Child Visits. Use the space under Matthew's name above and on the previous page to
record any relevant data. When you are finished, close Matthew's Chart and click on **Parent
Interview**. Observe both the **Health Supervision** and **Developmental Observations** sections
of the interview. As you observe Matthew and his father with the nurses, record any important
points above and on the previous page.

 Return to your textbook and read the sections on Cultural and Family Assessment in Chapter 2
on pp. 39-44.

3. Below and on the next page, complete a family and cultural assessment for Matthew and for
Sherrie. Base your assessment on what you have learned about each patient, using the
Friedman Family Assessment categories from Box 2-6 (p. 44) in your textbook as a guide.

Assessment Categories	Sherrie Bedonie	Matthew Brown
Family type		

Friedman Family Assessment

Affective function

Socialization function

Assessment Categories	Sherrie Bedonie	Matthew Brown
Reproductive function		
Economic function		
Health care function		
Cultural influences		
Values		
Health beliefs		
Religious influences		

4. How do the cultural and religious aspects of family influence the family structure for each of these children?

5. Why is it essential to include parents in all aspects of their child's health care?

6. Sherrie Bedonie has a stable two-parent family. How will this enhance her growth and development?

→ Return to the **Parent Interview** for Matthew Brown and observe the discussion between Matthew's father and the nurse practitioner.

7. Describe Matthew's family structure.

8. How should the nurse respond to Matthew's father when he talks about his wife?

9. What are some of the concerns expressed by Matthew's father?

10. What would you recommend to Matthew's father regarding supporting the parent-infant bonding process?

11. Based on Matthew's father's concerns, develop a nursing care plan below and on the next page. Write two priority nursing diagnoses and then provide short-term and long-term patient outcomes and nursing interventions to go with each diagnosis.

Nursing Diagnosis	Patient Outcomes	Nursing Interventions
a.	Short-term outcome:	

Nursing Diagnosis	Patient Outcomes	Nursing Interventions
	Long-term outcome:	
b.	Short-term outcome:	
	Long-term outcome:	

Return to your textbook and read about families with problems in Chapter 2 on pp. 32-35.

12. Families can become dysfunctional as a result of many factors. The inability to cope with stressful situations may cause conflict. For each of the areas below and on the next page, describe ways in which families under stress may not be able to cope.

Family Stressor	Description
Marital conflict or divorce	
Adolescent parenting	
Violence	

Family Stressor	Description
Substance abuse	
Child with special needs	

13. How can parents be assisted to cope with family stressors?

→ You will now visit two children who are in the Pediatric Unit and learn about their families. Return to the Nurses' Station and sign out of the current period by clicking on the **Login Computer**, selecting the **Supervisor's Computer** button, and then clicking on **Return to the Nurses' Station**. Now find the elevator and click to enter it. Take the elevator to the **Pediatric Unit (Floor 3)** by clicking **3** on the control panel to the right of the elevator door. When you arrive at Floor 3, click on the **Nurses' Station**. Sign in to visit Jason Baker in Room 306 at 11:00. He is a 14-year-old boy with diabetes who suffered a fractured leg in a basketball game. He is postoperative following surgery to reduce the fracture.

After listening to Jason's Case Overview, return to the Nurses' Station, click on **Patient Records**, and then click on **Chart**. Read about Jason's family in the History & Physical, Nursing History, and Admission Records in his Chart (keep notes below). Now return to the Nurses' Station and click on **Patient Care** and then on **Data Collection** on the drop-down menu. This will take you to the sink outside Jason's room (Room 306). After washing your hands, spend some time with Jason and his stepfather by clicking the **Behavior** button and then selecting each of the options under the photo of Jason. As you observe each video, keep notes in the space below.

Student Notes—Jason Baker's Family History

14. Using the history information you have gathered from Jason's Chart, draw a genogram of Jason's family below. (Use pp. 44 and 45 in your textbook as a guide.)

15. Describe the family relationship represented by the model you drew for question 14.

→ Now return to the Nurses' Station. (Wash your hands first!) Sign out from seeing Jason. (*Remember:* To do this, click on the **Supervisor's Computer** and then click on **Return to the Nurses' Station**.) Now sign in at 13:00 to see Kaylie Sern, age 3 years, who has been admitted for dehydration and otitis media. After reviewing Kaylie's Case Overview, click on **Patient Records** and then on **Chart**. Read the following sections of her Chart: History & Physical, Nursing History, and Admission Records. As you read, make notes below of any data regarding Kaylie's family history. Now return to the Nurses' Station and visit Kaylie and her family by clicking on **Patient Care** and then **Data Collection**. As always, wash your hands before entering the room. Once inside, click on the **Behavior** button and watch each of the videos, paying particular attention to the Activity section. Write down any important points below.

Student Notes—Kaylie Sern's Family History

16. What is the most important feature of Kaylie's family?

17. Using what you have learned from Kaylie's Chart, draw an ecomap of Kaylie's family below. (See pp. 44-45 in your textbook for help.)

18. Compare the relationships in Kaylie's family with those in Jason's family.

In your textbook read the section on Discipline on pp. 37-38 (Chapter 2) and the sections on Child Abuse and Neglect on pp. 1005-1012 (Chapter 30).

19. Parenting skills includes providing discipline. Discuss five different types of discipline techniques and the consequences of their use.

    a.

    b.

c.

d.

e.

20. What is the difference between abuse and neglect?

Abuse

Neglect

21. How should children be assessed for signs that they are victims of child abuse or neglect?

22. Below, identify two age groups of children who are most likely to be abused. Provide a rationale for why you chose each group.

    a.

    b.

23. Are any of the children you have visited today in the high-risk groups for child abuse or neglect? If so, who? What particular signs lead you (or *would* lead you) to suspect child abuse or neglect?

24. What are Kaylie's foster mother's concerns?

25. How could the nurse alleviate the anxiety Kaylie's parents are experiencing?

26. What is the legal procedure in your community regarding notifying authorities of suspected child abuse or neglect?

2

Communicating with Children and Families

Reading Assignment: Communicating with Children and Families (Chapter 3)

Patients: Matthew Brown, 10 months old, Well-Child Clinic, Room 205
Paul Parker, 24 months old, Well-Child Clinic, Room 202
Sherrie Bedonie, 4 years old, Well-Child Clinic, Room 204
De Olp, 6 years old, Pediatric Unit, Room 310

This clinical experience will focus on opportunities for you to observe and assess child/nurse and parent/nurse interactions in the Well-Child Clinic and the Pediatric Unit within the context of a nursing assessment. You will also critique the nurses' communication patterns within a developmental context. In this lesson, you will observe and compare communication styles and needs of children of various age groups during visits with an infant (Matthew Brown), a toddler (Paul Parker), a preschooler (Sherrie Bedonie), and a school-age child (De Olp). You will also be given the opportunity to critique these interactions and expand a nursing diagnosis to aid in the communication process among an ill child (De), her father, and the nurse.

Objectives

Upon completion of this lesson, you will be able to:

1. Describe communication.
2. Describe age-appropriate methods of nurse-patient communication.
3. Discuss nonverbal cues of communication.
4. Analyze parent/nurse communication in the well-child setting as it relates to anticipatory guidance.
5. Develop a nurse's aide orientation handout regarding communicating with ill children.
6. Critique nurse interactions with an ill child.
7. Develop patient outcomes and nursing interventions for this nursing diagnosis: Risk for impaired verbal communication for an ill child and her father.
8. Discuss how a nurse can best request that a parent return to the hospital because of a change in a child's physical condition.

In your textbook, read Chapter 3 about the different kinds of communication on pp. 50-52.

1. Based on what you have learned in your readings, in the chart below, give the best way to communicate in each of the age groups of children.

Communication Type	Infant	Toddler	Preschooler
Touch			
Physical Proximity			
Listening			
Visual			
Tone of Voice			
Body Language			

2. Why is touch so important to children?

In your textbook, read about family-centered communication in Chapter 3 on pp. 52-61.

CD-ROM Activity

Begin by going to the Well-Child Clinic (Floor 2), where you will visit three well children to observe communication between them, their parents, and the nurses. Go to the Nurses' Station, access the Login Computer, and sign in to see 24-month-old Paul Parker, who is at the clinic for his well-child visit. After listening to the Case Overview, visit Paul in Room 202 by clicking on **Physical Examination** in the upper left corner of your screen. Once inside the room, click on **Preliminary Examination** and then observe each section of the examination. As you watch and listen to each video, use the space below to record any particular findings relating to communication between Paul, his mother, and the nurse.

Student Notes—Physical Examination for Paul Parker

3. What did the nurse do (in terms of physical demeanor and proximity) that affected the data collection process?

4. How could the nurse have used play to enhance this nurse/child interaction?

5. Describe two situations in which the nurse directly asked Paul a question.

➡ Return to the Nurses' Station and click on **Parent Interview**. Then click on **Health Supervision** and observe the interactions between Paul's mother and the nurse practitioner.

6. Assess the body language of the mother during the parent interview.

7. How did inclusion of the mother enhance the situation?

8. Based on your observation of the mother, do you think she was comfortable speaking with the nurse? Explain.

➡ Return to the Nurses' Station. It is time for you to visit a different patient, so sign out from your visit with Paul Parker on the Login Computer. Now sign in to see Sherrie Bedonie, a 4-year-old girl who has her well-child appointment at 08:30 in Room 204. From the Nurses' Station, click on **Physical Examination**. Once inside the room, click on all assessment options to observe the entire examination, noticing the interactions among Sherrie, her mother, and the two nurses. Record your impressions of the communication exchanges below.

Student Notes—Physical Examination for Sherrie Bedonie

9. Review your notes from Sherrie's examination, as well as the notes you took earlier while observing Paul Parker's examination. Consider the interactions you observed during the various video segments. Below, list any similarities and differences you noticed between the communication processes of Paul and Sherrie during the videos.

Similarities between Paul and Sherrie

Differences between Paul and Sherrie

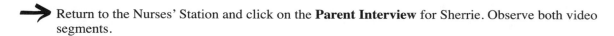 Return to the Nurses' Station and click on the **Parent Interview** for Sherrie. Observe both video segments.

10. In what ways did the nurse practitioner establish rapport with the mother during the Parent Interview?

11. Sherrie and her mother are Native Americans. Describe any specific cultural details you observed during the interaction with the nurse.

Return to the Nurses' Station and sign out from seeing Sherrie. Click again on the **Login Computer**, this time signing in to see Matthew Brown, a 10-month-old infant who is having an appointment at 10:00 in Room 205. From the Nurses' Station, click on **Parent Interview** and observe both segments of the video, paying attention to the interactions among Matthew, his father, and the nurse practitioner. Then return to the Nurses' Station and click on **Physical Examination**. (Wash your hands!) Once inside the room, observe Matthew's Physical Examination by clicking on the available assessment options. Write your impressions in the space provided below.

Student Notes—Physical Examination for Matthew Brown

12. How did the nurse practitioner use touch in the interview?

13. How would you describe the eye contact between the nurse practitioner and Matthew's father?

14. What type of communication did the nurse practitioner use with Matthew?

15. The nursing supervisor has asked you to create a handout that covers the issues involved in interacting with ill children. The handout will be used for an orientation class for the new nurses aides. Below, use any format you like to develop a handout that covers the concepts of effective communication. Review what you have learned from working with the three healthy children you just observed, and apply this knowledge to ill children, covering the following categories (at least). Use information from Table 3-3 (pp. 58-59), Table 3-4 (pp. 60-61), and Table 3-5 (p. 62) in your textbook to help add detail to your handout.

   a. Working with children

   b. Working with parents

   c. Using touch effectively

   d. Using play effectively

Communicating with Ill Children

➡ You will now go to the Pediatric Unit to observe communication between a nurse and an ill child. Return to the Nurses' Station and sign out. Then take the elevator to Floor 3. Go to the Nurses' Station and sign in at 11:00 to see De Olp, a 6-year-old girl in Room 310. De was diagnosed with acute lymphocytic leukemia on Saturday. Click on **Patient Records** and then on **Chart**. Inside De's Chart, review the Progress Notes since her admission. Pay particular attention to the subjective comments that De and her father made relating to her treatments over the past few days.

16. Critique the nurses' responses to De and her father's questions, as charted in the Progress Notes. Describe how you would have answered their questions.

17. As a first step in developing a new nursing care plan for De, provide patient outcomes and nursing interventions for the nursing diagnosis listed below.

Nursing Diagnosis	Patient Outcomes	Nursing Interventions
Risk for impaired verbal communication related to stress of patient and family regarding recent diagnosis		

➡ Now return to the Nurses' Station and click on **Patient Care** and **Data Collection**. (Wash your hands!) Once inside De's room, click on **Vital Signs** and then click on each of the assessment options, observing the interactions between De and the nurse during the vital signs measurements.

18. How does De's developmental level affect how the nurse speaks to her while taking vital signs?

→ Next, click on **Behavior** and watch those video segments.

19. Describe the interaction between the nurse, De, and her father.

→ Now take a virtual leap forward to a future time in De's hospitalization. Imagine that De's condition has suddenly deteriorated and she has been taken to the intensive care unit while her father is not in the hospital.

20. Write three sentences for a script to use when telling De's father about this serious change in his daughter's condition.

    a.

    b.

    c.

21. The scenario just described would be a stressful time for De and her father. Write a nursing care plan relating to the communication process for a child in poor health and family members.

Nursing Diagnosis	Patient Outcomes	Nursing Interventions

The Newborn

Reading Assignment: The Normal Newborn: Adaptation and Care (Chapter 5)
The Child with an Endocrine or Metabolic Alteration
(Chapter 28): Section on Inborn Errors of Metabolism

Patients: Matthew Brown, 10 months old, Well-Child Clinic, Room 205
Paul Parker, 24 months old, Well-Child Clinic, Room 202
Sherrie Bedonie, 4 years old, Well-Child Clinic, Room 204

In this lesson you will review the Charts of three well children and use their birth histories to describe particular aspects of newborn care. You will analyze newborn screening scores, plot birth measurements in a growth chart, describe newborn characteristics and testing methods, and develop a health teaching brochure for parents whose newborn is receiving phototherapy.

Objectives

Upon completion of this lesson, you will be able to:

1. Discuss various scoring systems that assess newborn health.
2. Use a growth chart.
3. Describe normal characteristics of newborns.
4. Discuss nursing interventions for newborns with meconium staining.
5. Provide health teaching for newborns receiving phototherapy.

CD-ROM Activity

Go to the Well-Child Clinic (Floor 2) to participate in a Chart audit on Matthew Brown, Sherrie Bedonie, and Paul Parker. When you arrive on Floor 2, click on the **Nurses' Station** and complete the following steps for each of the three children:
- Click on **Patient Records** and then on **Chart** in the drop-down menu.
- One at a time, click on and review the following sections: **Admissions Form**, **Birth & Health History**, **Growth Charts**, and **Laboratory Reports**.
- As you review each Chart section, record any data related to birth history and newborn characteristics in the space provided on the next page. (*Note:* Gather data on the birth history of Paul Parker's sister also.)
Remember: To switch from one patient to another, you will need to return to the Login Computer in the Nurses' Station, sign out for the current patient, and then sign in again for the next patient.

Student Notes—Chart Audit

	Matthew Brown	Sherrie Bedonie	Paul Parker	Paul's Sister
Admissions Form				

	Matthew Brown	Sherrie Bedonie	Paul Parker	Paul's Sister
Birth & Health History				

	Matthew Brown	Sherrie Bedonie	Paul Parker	Paul's Sister
Growth Charts and Laboratory Reports				

 Read pp. 98-124 in Chapter 5 of your textbook.

1. What is the normal range of values for each of the following vital signs in a newborn?

Respiratory rate

Heart rate

Temperature

2. What is an Apgar score?

3. List the five parts of the Apgar score.

   a.

   b.

   c.

   d.

   e.

4. What does it mean if a newborn has an Apgar score of 4 at 1 minute and a score of 6 at 5 minutes?

5. What is the New Ballard Score?

6. Below, list the signs to be assessed when using the New Ballard Score for the following categories.

Neuromuscular Maturity	Physical Maturity
a.	a.
b.	b.
c.	c.
d.	d.
e.	e.
f.	f.
	g.

7. From the newborn assessment findings in the Birth & Health History section of the Chart, list the Apgar and Ballard scores for each of the children below. Based on those scores, evaluate each child's health at birth.

Patient	Apgar Score	New Ballard Score	Evaluation
Matthew			
Paul			
Sherrie			

8. How and when should a newborn be weighed?

9. What points on a newborn's body are used as the starting and ending points when measuring that newborn's length?

10. During your Chart audit of Paul's history, you discovered that his birth weight, length, and head circumference were not plotted on the growth chart. On the growth chart provided on the next page, plot Paul's birth weight, birth length, and birth head circumference. Record the percentile ranking for each of these measurements in the Comment Section at the bottom of the chart.

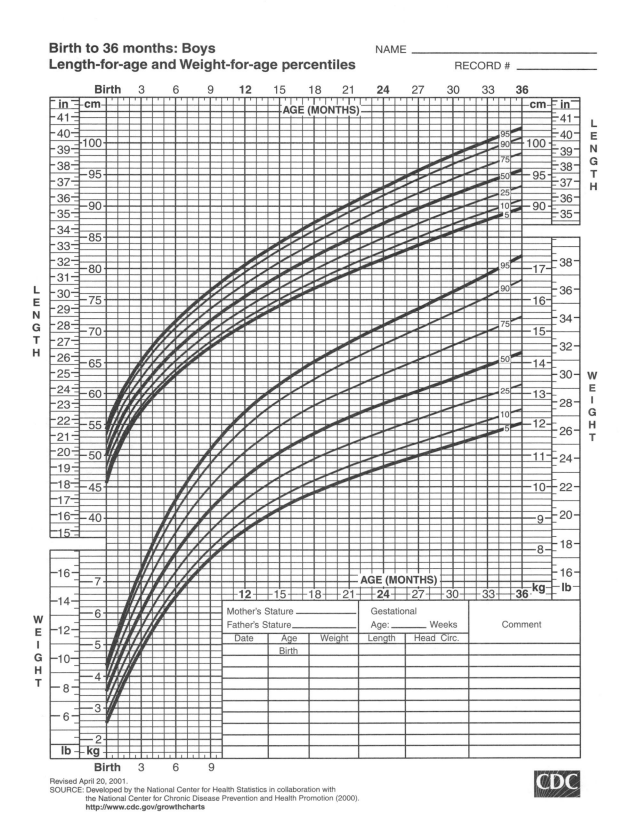

Birth to 36 months: Boys
Length-for-age and Weight-for-age percentiles

NAME _____

RECORD # _____

Revised April 20, 2001.
SOURCE: Developed by the National Center for Health Statistics in collaboration with
the National Center for Chronic Disease Prevention and Health Promotion (2000).
http://www.cdc.gov/growthcharts

CDC

11. Paul's history shows that his sister experienced a health problem during birth. Identify this problem and then list three nursing interventions to care for a newborn with this problem.

Problem

Interventions

12. List and describe six different newborn reflexes.

a.

b.

c.

d.

e.

f.

13. What recommendations would you make regarding the feeding of a newborn? Explain.

14. Discuss why Vitamin K (AquaMETHYTON) and optic antibiotics are given to newborn infants.

Vitamin K

Optic antibiotics

15. Both Paul and his sister have a history of breast-milk jaundice. Differentiate this type of jaundice from physiologic jaundice in regard to the following categories.

	Age at First Signs	Cause	Intervention
Breast-milk jaundice			
Physiologic jaundice			

16. List two nursing diagnoses and short-term patient outcomes for a newborn who is receiving phototherapy.

Nursing Diagnosis	**Short-Term Patient Outcome**

17. You have been asked to develop a standardized health teaching brochure to give to parents whose baby is to receive phototherapy at home. For each of the questions below, provide the necessary information for parents to know.

   a. What is phototherapy?

   b. What can my baby wear when receiving phototherapy?

   c. Why does my baby need eye patches?

   d. Can I take my baby out for feedings?

e. Why do I have to take my baby's temperature before feedings?

f. Why do I have to keep track of my baby's diaper changes?

18. The newborn teaching nurse has asked you to instruct a 21-year-old new mother about umbilical cord care for her newborn girl. Write a list of points that you want to emphasize to the mother in your teaching.

In your textbook, read about inborn errors of metabolism on pp. 905-912 in Chapter 28.

19. Newborn assessment also includes government-mandated testing to detect various treatable inborn errors of metabolism. Below, list the metabolism errors for which newborns are screened. Also describe each condition and provide the screening results for Matthew, Paul, and Sherrie.

Inborn Condition	Description	Matthew	Paul	Sherrie

The Infant

◠◠ **Reading Assignment:** Health Promotion for the Infant (Chapter 6)
Health Promotion for the Developing Child (Chapter 4): Section on Infants
Emergency Care of the Child (Chapter 11): Section on Lead Poisoning
The Child with a Hematologic Alteration (Chapter 24): Section on Iron Deficiency Anemia
Denver Developmental Screening Test II (Appendix F)

Patient: Matthew Brown, 10 months old, Well-Child Clinic, Room 205

This lesson focuses on understanding the growth and development of infants by simulating a well-child visit for a 10-month-old baby. The visit includes a developmental assessment from which you will conduct a Denver Developmental Screening Test II. Other issues related to infant immunizations, language, diet, play, and environmental safety are presented. You will also have the opportunity to plan care for an infant with iron deficiency anemia and to determine whether an infant is at risk for lead exposure.

Objectives

Upon completion of this lesson, you will be able to:

1. Carry out a developmental assessment for an infant.
2. Plan language-enhancing activities for an infant.
3. Select age-appropriate toys for an infant.
4. Analyze an infant's diet.
5. Discuss an infant's teeth.
6. Develop a health teaching plan regarding safety for families with an infant.
7. Discuss risk factors for infant lead exposure.

CD-ROM Activity

Go to the Well-Child Clinic on Floor 2. Once at the Nurses' Station, sign in to see Matthew Brown, a 10-month-old infant who is being seen in Room 205 at 10:00.

Review Matthew's history by clicking on **Patient Records**, then on **Chart**, and then on the following sections: **Birth & Health History**, **Immunization Record**, **Well-Child Visits**, **Sick-Child Visits**, and **Growth Charts**. Write any notes of particular interest in the space below.

Student Notes

Birth & Health History

Immunization Record

Well-Child Visits

Sick-Child Visits

Growth Charts

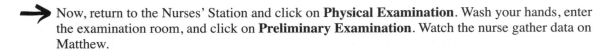 Now, return to the Nurses' Station and click on **Physical Examination**. Wash your hands, enter the examination room, and click on **Preliminary Examination**. Watch the nurse gather data on Matthew.

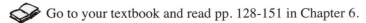 Go to your textbook and read pp. 128-151 in Chapter 6.

1. Comparing Matthew's current weight, height, and head circumference with the measurements already recorded on his growth charts, how would you describe his growth?

2. What is the rule of thumb regarding expected weight gain and growth in length for infants based on their birth weight and length?

3. Is Matthew on target for his weight and length at this 10-month well-child visit? (*Hint:* You need to convert his current weight from kilograms to pounds first to make the comparison. Show all of your work in the space below.)

4. Matthew's Chart shows that he is up to date on all of his immunizations. Below, match the name of each vaccination Matthew has received with the corresponding disease(s) against which the vaccination protects him.

_____ Hep B   a. Measles, mumps, rubella

_____ DTaP   b. Chickenpox

_____ Hib   c. Pneumococcal disease

_____ IPV   d. Hepatitis B

_____ MMR   e. Diphtheria, tetanus, pertussis

_____ Varicella   f. Polio

_____ PCV (Prevnar)   g. *Haemophilus influenzae* type b

5. In anticipation of Matthew's next well-child visit, at which time he is due to receive his 12-month DTaP vaccine, what should the nurse plan to teach his father about this next immunization?

Return to the Nurses' Station and click on **Parent Interview** and then on **Developmental Observations**. Take notes below on what you observe during this interview. Then return to the Nurses' Station and click on **Developmental Surveillance** to review Matthew's developmental assessment. Record important points in the space below.

Student Notes

 Now refer to Chapter 4 (pp. 79-83 and 1073-1074) in your textbook and the section on Assessment of Development. This reading introduces another screening test that could be done with Matthew—the Denver Developmental Screening Test II (DDST-II).

6. On the Denver II chart on the next page, draw a vertical line at 10 months for Matthew's age. For each skill intersecting his age line, place a Pass or Fail mark, comparing the findings of Matthew's 9-month developmental screening with this DDST-II. Are the findings comparable? Provide rationales for your answers.

Denver II

Examiner:
Date:

Name:
Birthdate:
ID No.:

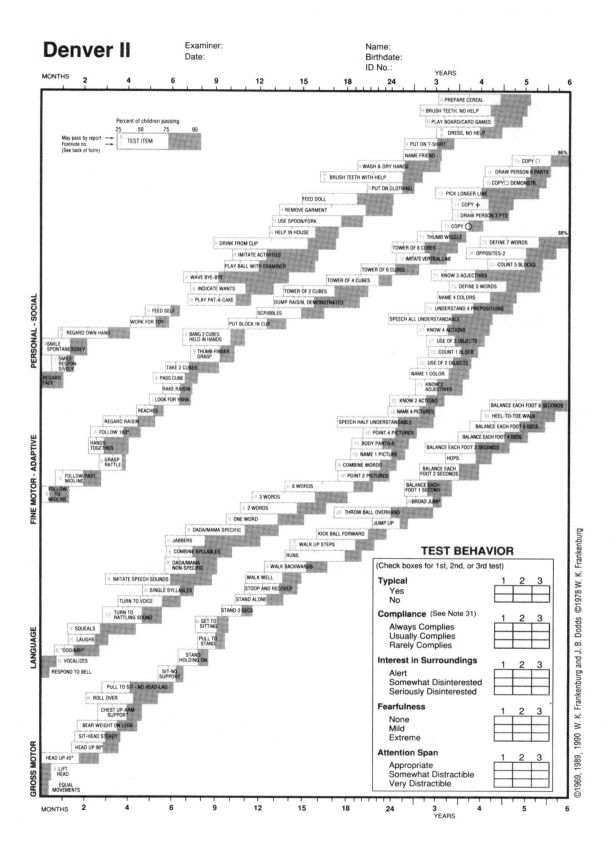

Review the developmental theories of Piaget, Erikson, and Freud regarding infants in Chapter 4 (pp. 69-73 and Table 4-1) of your textbook.

7. Based on Matthew's achievement of the specific developmental tasks identified by each of the theorists listed below, indicate Matthew's current stage in each theoretical model. Also describe the focus of each of these stages.

Theorist	Stage	Focus
Piaget		
Freud		
Erikson		

8. How do the infant milestones described by the developmental theories in question 7 affect the health care that Matthew receives?

9. Based on your observation of the interactions between Matthew, his father, and the nurse practitioner, how would you assess Matthew's language development?

10. Since Matthew's father is concerned about his son's speech, what recommendations would you make to help Matthew continue to develop his language skills?

11. List seven kinds of toys that the nurse should recommend for Matthew to play with.

    a.

    b.

    c.

    d.

    e.

    f.

    g.

12. What diet did Matthew's father say Matthew has been eating? Analyze the appropriateness of this diet for a 10-month-old infant.

In your textbook, read the section on iron deficiency anemia on pp. 744-746 in Chapter 24.

13. What is iron deficiency anemia, and why does it occur?

14. What makes an infant susceptible to developing iron deficiency anemia?

15. Why is supplemental iron an essential part of Matthew's diet? If Matthew were suspected of having iron deficiency anemia, what nursing assessment findings would be seen?

16. Give six nursing interventions used to care for infants with iron deficiency anemia.

    a.

    b.

    c.

    d.

    e.

    f.

17. Matthew eats some solid baby foods. Below, rank the foods listed in the left column in the order in which they should be tried with infants who are beginning to eat solids. For each food group, provide two specific examples.

Rank for Starting	Food Examples
_____ Fruits	(1)
	(2)
_____ Vegetables	(1)
	(2)
_____ Cereals	(1)
	(2)

18. At 10 months, Matthew probably has been attempting to feed himself. Based on this assumption, what safety measures should be used during feeding time?

19. Matthew was assessed as having teeth. Rank the usual order in which the following deciduous teeth appear in infants.

    _____ Molars

    _____ Canines

    _____ Upper central incisors

    _____ Lower lateral incisors

    _____ Upper lateral incisors

    _____ Lower central incisors

20. Teaching the parents about the teething process should include what four categories of information?

    a.

    b.

    c.

    d.

21. When should Matthew begin dental hygiene?

22. Bottle mouth caries are sometimes a health problem for older infants who have teeth. Give the appropriate nursing diagnosis, patient outcome, and nursing intervention for this potential problem.

Nursing Diagnosis	Patient Outcome	Nursing Intervention

→ Return to the Nurses' Station, click on **Anticipatory Guidance**, and review Matthew's checklists.

23. Develop a health teaching plan for all of Matthew's caretakers that focuses on environmental safety for Matthew in each of the categories listed below and on the next page.

Category	Information to Include in Health Teaching Plan
Water safety	
Home safety	

Category	Information to Include in Health Teaching Plan

Motor vehicle safety

Return to your textbook and read about lead poisoning on p. 292 in Chapter 11.

24. Why should older infants be screened for lead ingestion?

25. What three questions should the nurse ask Matthew's father to determine whether Matthew is at high risk for lead exposure?

    a.

    b.

    c.

26. For each question you wrote above, provide an answer that would indicate a child was indeed at risk for lead exposure.

    a.

    b.

    c.

The Toddler

📖 **Reading Assignment:** Health Promotion for the Developing Child (Chapter 4):
Sections on Toddlers
Health Promotion During Early Childhood (Chapter 7)
Denver Developmental Screening Test II (Appendix F)

Patient: Paul Parker, 24 months old, Well-Child Clinic, Room 202

This lesson focuses on health promotion during the toddler period (roughly ages 1 year through 3 years). You will visit Paul Parker, a 24-month-old boy who is receiving a well-child check-up. Areas of study in this lesson include growth and development, nutrition, preparation for toilet training, play, and discipline for toddlers. This visit also contains a developmental assessment from which you will conduct a Denver Developmental Screening Test II.

Objectives

Upon completion of this lesson, you will be able to:

1. Analyze growth rates in the toddler.
2. Analyze different developmental theories as they apply to toddlers.
3. Carry out a Denver Developmental Screening Test II for a toddler.
4. Plan a nursing care plan and speech development activities for a toddler.
5. Develop a brochure regarding readiness of a toddler for toilet training.
6. Analyze a toddler's diet and prepare a 2-day menu.
7. Select age-appropriate toys for a toddler.
8. Discuss toddler discipline.
9. Provide recommendations regarding safety for toddlers.

CD-ROM Activity

For this lesson, you will again work in the Well-Child Clinic (Floor 2). Once in the Nurses' Station, access the Login Computer and sign in for Paul Parker (Room 202) at 07:00. Click on **Patient Records** on the left side of the screen. Within Paul's Chart, review the following sections: Birth & Health History, Well-Child Visits, Sick-Child Visits, Developmental Surveillance, Growth Charts, and Referral Forms. Write down any important points that you want to remember in the space provided on the next page.

Student Notes—Paul Parker's Chart Review

Birth & Health History

Well-Child Visits

Sick-Child Visits

Developmental Surveillance

Growth Charts

Referral Forms

Go to your textbook and read the material related to toddlers on pp. 154-158 and p. 160.

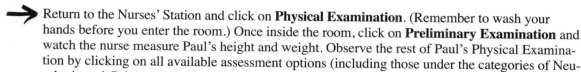 Return to the Nurses' Station and click on **Physical Examination**. (Remember to wash your hands before you enter the room.) Once inside the room, click on **Preliminary Examination** and watch the nurse measure Paul's height and weight. Observe the rest of Paul's Physical Examination by clicking on all available assessment options (including those under the categories of Neurologic and Gait, as well as those accessed by clicking on the various parts of the body model).

1. What is the general rule of thumb regarding estimates of toddler height and weight based on birth measurements?

Height

Weight

2. What are Paul's height and weight now?

3. Find Paul's birth height and weight. (*Hint:* Check his Birth & History.) Comparing these measurements to his present size, how would you assess his growth? (*Hint:* You need to convert pounds to kilograms to make the comparison.)

 In your textbook, read pp. 69-74 on the developmental theories for toddlers.

4. In the chart below and on the next page, identify the primary focus of development for toddlers, according to each of the theorists listed. For each focus, provide a specific example.

Theorist	Focus for Toddlers	Example
Piaget		
Freud		

Theorist	Focus for Toddlers	Example
Erikson		
Kohlberg		

5. Based on these four theoretical frameworks, how do you expect Paul to behave during the upcoming assessment?

Return to your textbook and review pp. 79-83 in Chapter 4 and pp. 1073-1074 in Appendix F.

You will now conduct a developmental assessment of Paul. Refer to the information you gathered from his Developmental Surveillance and recorded on p. 88 of this lesson. If necessary, click on Developmental Surveillance from the Nurses' Station and review as needed to compare his past and present development.

6. What are the findings regarding Paul's current development?

7. The Denver Developmental Screening Test II (DDST-II) is another tool that could be used to assess Paul Parker's development. On the DDST-II sheet on the next page, draw a vertical line at the 2-year age mark and write in Paul's behavior in each of the categories. For each skill intersecting his age line, place a Pass or Fail mark, comparing the findings of Paul's 24-month developmental screening with this DDST-II.

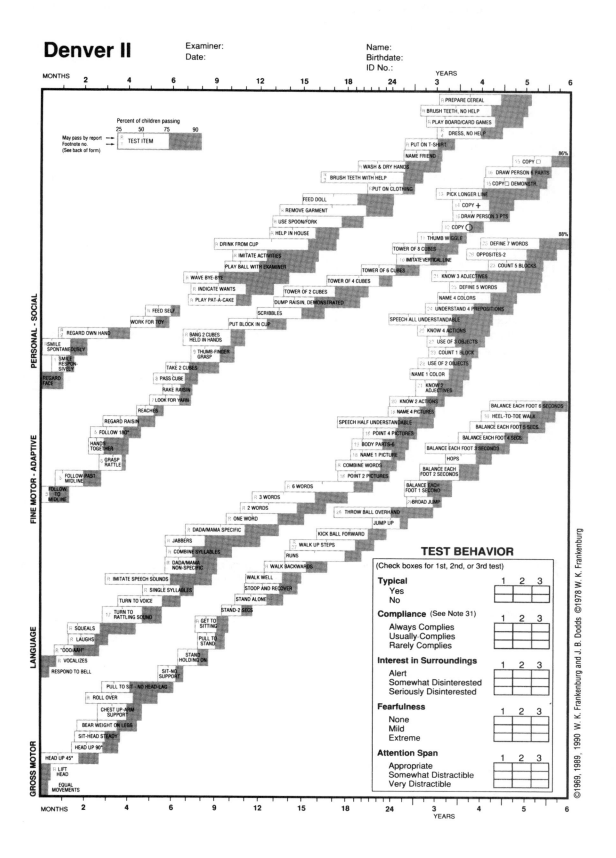

8. Compared with the nurse practitioner's assessment summary of findings in the Developmental Surveillance, how does Paul fare in the DDST-II?

In your textbook, read the section pertaining to the toddler on p. 159.

9. Compare Paul's speech ability with the expected language development for a toddler.

10. Does Paul appear to have a speech deficit? _____ Below, give the appropriate nursing diagnosis, patient outcome, and nursing interventions to help guide nursing care for a toddler with a speech deficit.

Nursing Diagnosis	Patient Outcome	Nursing Interventions

Return to the Nurses' Station and click on **Parent Interview**. View both the Health Supervision and Developmental Observations segments. Make note of any important points in the space below.

Student Notes

Health Supervision

Developmental Observations

Review pp. 173-174 and Box 7-8 in your textbook.

11. Because Paul is 24 months old, his mother may be concerned about beginning toilet training. Is Paul ready for toilet training? Explain your answer.

12. The nurse has asked you to draw a poster for the waiting room that helps parents recognize whether a toddler is ready for toilet training. Create such a poster below.

Return to Chapter 4 (pp. 89-92) and Chapter 7 (pp. 165-166) in your textbook and read the sections on nutrition for toddlers.

13. Paul's mother is concerned about his eating. What are Paul's current eating habits and preferences? (*Hint:* Use your notes from the Parent Interview. If necessary, replay the video.) What three examples of guidance can you provide Paul's mother about his eating habits?

    a.

    b.

    c.

14. What is the term generally used to denote a toddler's feeding resistance?

15. Write an appropriate 2-day menu plan for Paul, including breakfast, lunch, dinner, and snacks. (*Hint:* Refer to Figure 4-5 (p. 91) in Chapter 4 of your textbook.)

Meal	Day #1	Day #2
Breakfast		
Lunch		
Dinner		
Snacks		

In your textbook, review pp. 162-163 in Chapter 7 and pp. 83-86 in Chapter 4.

16. What type of play activities are normally seen in toddlers? Describe these in detail.

17. What five types of toys would you recommend for Paul?

    a.

    b.

    c.

    d.

    e.

 Read pp. 160-162, 168-170, and 174 in your textbook.

18. How does Paul's mother describe his behavior at home? (*Hint:* Use your notes from the Parent Interview.)

19. Describe how parents can deal with this behavior.

20. Why do toddlers exhibit this behavior?

21. Discuss how negativism and ritualism in toddlers influences their behavior.

Negativism

Ritualism

22. Sleep is important for toddlers. What are Paul's usual sleep habits? (*Hint:* Refer to Parent Interview video or your notes.) What would you recommend regarding naps and sleeping for Paul?

Return to your textbook and read pp. 170-171.

Return to the Nurses' Station, click on **Anticipatory Guidance**, and review Paul's checklists.

23. Considering that Paul is an active toddler, what safety recommendations would you make for each of the following categories?

Safety Category	Recommendations for Paul
Motor vehicle safety	
Poisoning prevention	

24. Provide anticipatory guidance for the following issues related to teaching hygiene to toddlers.

    a. Teaching handwashing

    b. Teaching dental hygiene

The Preschooler

👓 **Reading Assignment:** Health Promotion for the Developing Child (Chapter 4):
Sections for Preschoolers
Health Promotion During Early Childhood (Chapter 7):
Sections for Preschoolers
Denver Developmental Screening Test II (Appendix F)

Patient: Sherrie Bedonie, 4 years old, Well-Child Clinic, Room 204

This lesson focuses on preschoolers, children between the ages of 3 and 6 years. You will conduct a well-child visit for a preschool girl, 4-year-old Sherrie Bedonie, and observe the assessment for growth and development. Opportunities are provided for you to conduct a Denver Developmental Screening Test II, develop a nursing care plan regarding play, and devise health teaching plans about snacks. Dental care, safety, and school readiness are also covered in this lesson.

Objectives

Upon completion of this lesson, you will be able to:

1. Analyze growth rates in the preschooler.
2. Differentiate among several developmental theories relating to preschooler development.
3. Carry out a developmental assessment for a preschooler.
4. Select age-appropriate toys for a preschooler.
5. Develop a nursing care plan regarding play for a preschooler.
6. Discuss dental hygiene for the preschooler.
7. Analyze a preschooler's diet.
8. Write a health teaching plan regarding school readiness.

💿 CD-ROM Activity

Go to the Well-Child Clinic on Floor 2. Once in the Nurses' Station, sign in to see 4-year-old Sherrie Bedonie at 08:30 in Room 204. Click on **Patient Records** to open Sherrie's Chart. review the following sections: Birth & Health History, Well-Child Visits, Sick-Child Visits, Developmental Surveillance, and Growth Charts. Write down any important points that you want to remember in the space provided on the next page.

Student Notes—Sherrie Bedonie's Chart Review

Birth & Health History

Well-Child Visits

Sick-Child Visits

Developmental Surveillance

Growth Charts

In your textbook, read pp. 156 and 158-159 in Chapter 7.

→ Return to the Nurses' Station and click on **Physical Examination**. After washing your hands, enter the examination room and observe the Preliminary Examination. After watching the nurse collect data in all categories of the Preliminary Examination, click on the head of the 3-D body model and observe all segments of the Head & Neck Examination. Next, click on **Vital Signs**, and watch the nurse as she measures Sherrie's weight and height.

1. What are Sherrie's height and weight?

2. Based on what you found in the Growth Charts section of Sherrie's Chart, how would you assess her growth pattern? (*Hint:* Use the chart for girls, 2 to 20 years.)

Review the developmental theories of Piaget, Freud, Erikson, and Kohlberg as they relate to the preschool child in Chapter 4 (pp. 69-74) of your textbook.

3. In the chart below, identify the primary focus of preschoolers' thinking, according to each of the theorists listed. For each focus, provide a specific example.

Theorist	Focus for Preschoolers	Example
Piaget		
Freud		
Erikson		
Kohlberg		

4. Based on Piaget's theory on preschoolers' thinking, explain why Sherrie brought toys with her to the clinic.

5. Freud's theory discusses the Oedipus/Electra complex in preschoolers. Explain this complex and discuss how Sherrie may behave relating to this theory.

6. What is magical thinking?

7. How might Sherrie show this behavior?

8. Children in the preschool age group also begin to exhibit sexual curiosity. What would you recommend to Sherrie's mother regarding this?

➤ From the Nurses' Station, click on **Developmental Surveillance** and review Sherrie's checklists. Then return to the Nurses' Station and click on **Parent Interview**. Observe both the Health Supervision and Developmental Observations segments of the interview.

9. What were the findings of the Developmental Surveillance?

Return to your textbook and read pp. 79-83 in Chapter 4 and pp. 1073-1074 in Appendix F.

10. Another tool that could be used to assess Sherrie's development is the Denver Developmental Screening Test II (DDST-II). On the DDST-II sheet on the next page, draw a vertical line at the 4-year age mark and record Sherrie's behavior in each of the categories based on her own developmental assessment. For each skill intersecting her age line, place a Pass or Fail mark, comparing the findings of Sherrie's 4-year developmental screening with this DDST-II.

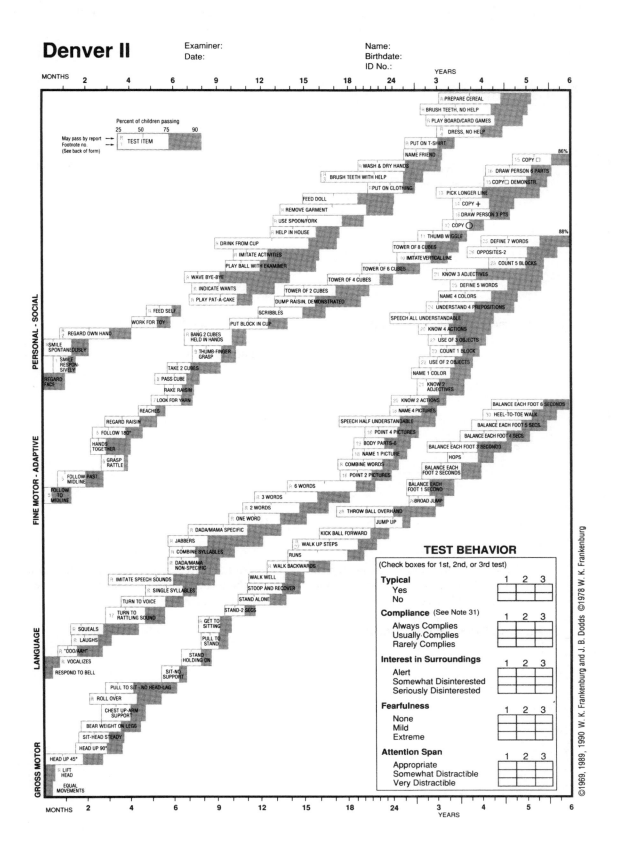

Denver II

11. Compared to the nurse practitioner's assessment (in the Developmental Surveillance), how does Sherrie fare in the DDST-II? Provide a rationale for your answer.

12. How would you describe Sherrie's home life? What should the nurse expect to find when assessing her play?

Read about preschoolers on pp. 83-85 and 162-165 in your textbook.

13. List six toys or activities that would be appropriate for Sherrie.

    a.

    b.

    c.

    d.

    e.

    f.

14. Because Sherrie has little interaction with children her own age, the nurse practitioner asks you to develop a nursing care plan to help focus the health teaching of Sherrie's mother regarding Sherrie's play. In the boxes below, complete the care plan.

Nursing Diagnosis	Short-Term Outcome	Nursing Interventions

Read pp. 165-167 in Chapter 7 of your textbook.

15. What observations were made about Sherrie's teeth? What health teaching should be given regarding Sherrie's dental hygiene? (*Hint:* Refer to the notes you took of Sherrie's Well-Child Visits regarding her teeth.)

16. Sherrie's mother is concerned about Sherrie eating between meals. Name six snacks that would be appropriate for Sherrie to eat.

    a.

    b.

    c.

    d.

    e.

    f.

17. Using Figure 4-5 on p. 91 in your textbook, review the snack recommendations you made in question 16. List three other appropriate choices to ensure proper nutrition regarding Sherrie's snack choices.

18. Sherrie sometimes misbehaves. What type of discipline would you recommend for Sherrie?

19. Based on Sherrie's weight and recommended motor vehicle safety guidelines, circle the type of car restraint she should be using from the choices below. Provide a rationale for your answer. (*Hint:* You need to convert Sherrie's present weight from kilograms to pounds first to complete this question.)

    Car seat   Booster seat   Seat belt

    Rationale:

20. List and discuss four types of safety other than motor vehicle safety that the nurse practitioner should go over with Sherrie's mother.

Safety Topic	**Discussion**
a.	
b.	
c.	
d.	

Read pp. 176-178 in your textbook.

21. The nurse practitioner anticipates that Sherrie may not be ready for kindergarten next year, so she asks you to develop a health teaching sheet for the mother to follow to help Sherrie prepare for school. Develop your teaching sheet below.

The School-Age Child

_____

∽⚭ **Reading Assignment:** Health Promotion for the School-Age Child (Chapter 8)
Health Promotion for the Developing Child (Chapter 4):
Sections for School-Age Children

Patients: De Olp, 6 years old, Pediatric Unit, Room 310
Maria Ortiz, 8 years old, Pediatric Unit, Room 308

In this lesson, you will be introduced to De Olp, a 6-year-old girl diagnosed with acute lympho-cytic leukemia. You will focus on the growth and developmental components of the healthy school-age child by reviewing the theories of growth and development, play, nutrition, dental care, and safety through extrapolation of data from De's Chart. Particular attention is paid to the major adjustment of going to school and the stressors affecting children in this age group. You will then have the opportunity to compare De's development with that of Maria Ortiz, an 8-year-old who was admitted to the pediatric unit for asthma. Development of a health teaching plan to teach sex education to school-age children is also included in this lesson.

Objectives

Upon completion of this lesson, you will be able to:

1. Analyze the growth rate of a school-age girl.
2. Differentiate among several developmental theories relating to the school-age child's development.
3. Describe the play activities of the school-age child.
4. Develop a 2-day menu for a school-age child based on the Food Guide Pyramid.
5. Discuss dental changes in the school-age child.
6. Discuss prevention of injuries in the school-age child.
7. Describe the effects of going to school.
8. Discuss recommendations to help alleviate stressors in the school-age child.
9. Write a health teaching sheet about sex education for elementary school students.

⚬ CD-ROM Activity

For this lesson, you will be working in the Pediatric Unit (Floor 3). Proceed to the Floor 3 Nurses' Station and sign in to see 6-year-old De Olp at 07:00 (Room 310). Return to the Nurses' Station and click on **Patient Records** and then on **Chart** in the drop-down menu. Within De's Chart, read the following sections: History & Physical, Nursing History, and Admissions Records. Write down any important points about her growth and development in the space provided on the next page.

➜ **Student Notes—De Olp's Chart Review**

History & Physical

Nursing History

Admissions Records

 Read pp. 182-184 relating to the school-age child in Chapter 8 of your textbook.

1. What is the usual rate of weight gain and height increase per year during the school-age years?

Weight gain

Height increase

2. What are De's height and weight?

3. Referring to the growth chart for girls ages 2 to 20 years on the next page, how would you assess De's growth pattern?

2 to 20 years: Girls
Stature-for-age and Weight-for-age percentiles

NAME _____

RECORD # _____

Date	Age	Weight	Stature	BMI*

Mother's Stature _____   Father's Stature _____

To Calculate BMI: Weight (kg) ÷ Stature (cm) ÷ Stature (cm) x 10,000
or Weight (lb) ÷ Stature (in) ÷ Stature (in) x 703

AGE (YEARS)

Revised and corrected November 21, 2000.
SOURCE: Developed by the National Center for Health Statistics in collaboration with
the National Center for Chronic Disease Prevention and Health Promotion (2000).
http://www.cdc.gov/growthcharts

CDC

Review the developmental theories of Piaget, Freud, Erikson, and Kohlberg in Chapter 4 of your textbook (pp. 69-74). Then read pp. 184-199 in Chapter 8 as they relate to the school-age child.

4. In the chart below, identify the primary focus of school-age children's thinking, according to each theorist listed. For each focus, provide a specific example.

Theorist	Focus for School-Age Children	Example
Piaget		
Freud		
Erikson		
Kohlberg		

5. Based on the fact that De is 6 years old, how should the nurse use knowledge about De's developmental level in giving nursing care?

6. What should the nurse anticipate about De's use of language?

7. What four types of play activities would De most likely engage in at home?

   a.

   b.

   c.

   d.

8. De will probably make some friends while she is in the hospital. Why is this anticipated?

9. Going to school is the most important part of a school-age child's life. Knowing that De is a first grader, what would you predict are her feelings about school?

10. As the nurse, what would you recommend if De's father told you that De hates school?

11. If De were experiencing anxiety regarding school (school refusal), what signs would most likely be seen?

12. De is an only child, and her father works full-time. As the nurse, what would you recommend regarding her after-school time since being left alone after school may constitute parental neglect in her community?

13. De indicates that she eats three meals per day plus snacks. Devise a 2-day menu plan for De, using the food category guidelines cited on p. 188 of your textbook. First, write the food categories and number of servings required on the pyramid below. Then, under each day's heading, list the specific foods that De will eat on that day.

Day 1   **Day 2**

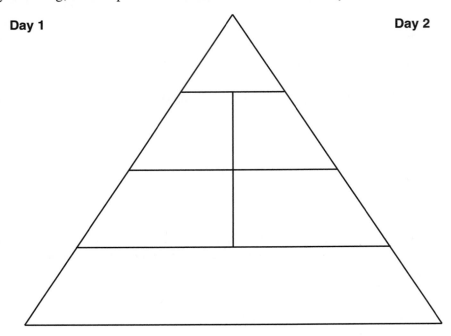

→ Return to the Nurses' Station and click on **Patient Care** and then on **Data Collection** on the drop-down menu. Wash your hands and enter De's room. Once inside, click on the head of the body model. This reveals assessment options for the Head & Neck examination. Click on **EENT** and watch the nurse's assessment of De's mouth.

14. Although there is no information related to De's teeth in the Chart, what would you expect to find during an assessment of De's mouth?

15. Which baby teeth are usually lost first?

16. What three recommendations should be made regarding dental care for a healthy 6-year-old?

   a.

   b.

   c.

17. How much sleep does a 6-year-old need?

18. Comparing your answer to question 17 with De's sleep history as documented in the Nursing History section of her Chart, what would you recommend regarding her sleep patterns?

19. What type of discipline works best for a school-age child?

20. Safety is an important issue for school-age children. Based on the following nursing diagnosis for a healthy school-age child, list long-term patient outcomes and nursing interventions relating to safety.

Nursing Diagnosis	Long-Term Patient Outcomes	Nursing Interventions
Risk for injury related to developmental age		

It is time for you to visit another patient on this floor. Return to the Nurses' Station and sign out from De's care. Then reenter the Login Computer and sign in to see Maria Ortiz in Room 308 at 09:00. Maria is an 8-year-old girl who has been admitted for an acute asthmatic episode. From the Nurses' Station click on **Patient Records** and then **Chart**. Within Maria's Chart, click on the **Nursing History** tab. Referring again to the elements of growth and development for school-age children, review Maria's overall pattern of growth so far. Write any important points in the space provided below.

Student Notes—Maria Ortiz' Chart Review

21. Based on a review of the theoretical concepts you covered relating to school-age children in question 4 of this lesson, how is 8-year-old Maria different in her cognitive development from 6-year-old De?

22. Listed below and on the next page are common sources of stress for school-age children. For each source of stress, indicate with a Y or an N whether or not it is likely to be a problem for Maria. For each source that applies to Maria, write recommendations that you would give Maria and her mother to help them cope.

Sources of Stress	Applies to Maria (Y/N)	Recommendations
School pressures		
Physical threats		

Sources of Stress	Applies to Maria (Y/N)	Recommendations
Competitive sports		
Activity overload		
Family pressures		
Media influence		

23. At age 8 years, Maria may be exhibiting curiosity about sex and "where babies come from." Since sex education is now recommended to begin for children in elementary school, develop an outline below, listing the topics that should be covered in a sex education class for a third-grade class.

24. What methods would you use to conduct a sex education health teaching class for third-grade children?

The Adolescent

Reading Assignment: Health Promotion for the Adolescent (Chapter 9)
Health Promotion for the Developing Child: Sections for the
Adolescent (Chapter 4)

Patient: Jason Baker, 14 years old, Pediatric Unit, Room 306

The aspects of growth and development of the early male adolescent are the focus of this lesson. You will be introduced to 14-year-old Jason Baker, who is recovering from surgery to repair his fractured leg. Despite Jason's injury, this lesson will focus only on issues related to the *healthy* teenager. You will have the opportunity to conduct theoretical and practice-based investigations related to the physical and cognitive changes in adolescents, their nutritional needs, and the reduction of risk as related to injury prevention, gang involvement, suicide, and sex education.

Objectives

Upon completion of this lesson, you will be able to:

1. Plot an adolescent's weight on a growth chart.
2. Differentiate adolescent growth spurts for boys and girls.
3. Identify pubertal changes in adolescent boys.
4. Differentiate among several developmental theories relating to the adolescent's development.
5. Discuss recreational activities of adolescents.
6. Develop "teenager-friendly" food substitutes for junk food.
7. Write an educational brochure on injury prevention.
8. Plan a presentation regarding prevention of gang involvement.
9. Analyze an adolescent's suicide risk.
10. Develop a nursing care plan regarding provision of sex education for adolescents.

CD-ROM Activity

For this lesson, you will continue working on the Pediatric Unit (Floor 3). Go to the Floor 3 Nurses' Station and sign in to see 14-year-old Jason Baker (Room 306) at 05:30. Read the Assignment in the Course Overview; then return to the Nurses' Station. Click on **Patient Records** and then **Chart** in the drop-down menu. Once inside Jason's Chart, read his History & Physical, Nursing History, and Admissions Records. Make note of any important points about his growth and development in the space provided on the next page.

Student Notes—Jason Baker's Chart Review

History & Physical

Nursing History

Admissions Records

Go to your textbook and review pp. 204-209 in Chapter 9.

1. Adolescence is a time of many physical changes. For each of the two changes listed below, indicate the age at which the change occurs for boys and for girls.

Changes	Boys	Girls
Growth spurt		
Secondary sex characteristics		

2. Based on the information you gathered from Jason's Chart, plot his weight on the Growth Chart provided on the next page. Assess Jason's growth at this time.

2 to 20 years: Boys
Stature-for-age and Weight-for-age percentiles

NAME _____

RECORD # _____

Mother's Stature _____ Father's Stature _____

Date	Age	Weight	Stature	BMI*

*To Calculate BMI: Weight (kg) ÷ Stature (cm) ÷ Stature (cm) x 10,000
or Weight (lb) ÷ Stature (in) ÷ Stature (in) x 703

AGE (YEARS)

3. What is the Tanner Scale?

4. Although Jason's genitourinary examination was deferred, at what stage of the Tanner scale would the nurse expect him to be at his age (14 years)?

→ Return to the Nurses' Station and click on **Patient Care** and then on **Data Collection**. Wash your hands and then click on the curtain to the right of the sink. This takes you to the Pre-Op Interview. Click on **View Interview** and observe the interactions and communication exchange between Jason and the surgical nurse.

5. Critique the nurse's discussion with Jason. Was it developmentally appropriate? Explain.

6. Listen to Jason's voice during his interactions with the nurse. How would you assess the quality of his voice?

Review the developmental theories of Piaget, Freud, Erikson, and Kohlberg, as they relate to the adolescent, in Chapter 4 (pp. 69-74) and Chapter 9 (pp. 209-213) of your textbook.

7. In the chart below and on the next page, identify the primary focus of adolescent thinking, according to each of the listed theorists. For each focus, provide a specific example.

Theorist	Focus for Adolescents	Example
Piaget		

Theorist	Focus for Adolescents	Example
Freud		
Erikson		
Kohlberg		

8. How would you expect Jason to interact with others, based on his level of cognitive development?

9. Since Jason, at age 14 years, is in early adolescence, what types of activities would the nurse anticipate that he enjoys? How does this compare with findings in Jason's Nursing History?

10.   What is the "imaginary audience"? How does this relate to adolescent functioning?

Return to your textbook and read pp. 213-221.

11. Because of the vast physical changes that occur during adolescence, nutritional needs may not always be met. Below, create a junk food diet that may be typical for many adolescents. Then, in the right column, replace each junk food item with a nutritional, yet "teenager-friendly" food. (*Hint:* Remember from Jason's History & Physical that he also has diabetes. Review nutritional guidelines for adolescents with diabetes on pp. 927 and 932 if you wish.)

Meal	Junk Food	Nutritional Alternative Food
Breakfast		
Lunch		
Dinner		
Snacks		

12. What is the major dental milestone in teenagers?

13. What dental information were you able to obtain from Jason's Chart assessment?

14. Jason's school nurse has asked you to summarize the concepts of adolescent invulnerability (personal fable) and injury prevention for a brochure to be distributed in Jason's middle school, specifically to his eighth-grade class. Since injuries account for the majority of adolescent deaths—and you want the brochure to be as complete as possible—which topics related to safety should be included? Develop an outline for the brochure below, making sure to include those topics about safety.

15. Peer relationships are important for adolescents. Based on what you learned from Jason's Nursing History, how would you assess his social relationships?

16. Your clinical instructor has asked you to give a 10-minute presentation to the parent-teacher organization of Jason's middle school, focusing on prevention of gang development in the community. What should you include in your talk? Outline your presentation below.

17. What would be your response if Jason told you that sometimes he feels as if life is not worth living?

18. Jason's mother calls you, frantically telling you that Jason wants to dye his hair green and get a tattoo of his basketball team's mascot on his arm when he gets home from the hospital. She said that she went along with Jason's wishes when he had his ears pierced, but that this is too much. What recommendation could you make to his mother?

19. Suppose Jason tells you that he is concerned that he is missing his sex education classes at school and says that he has some questions. What topics would you anticipate he has questions about? How would you handle the discussion? Develop a nursing care plan below to guide your discussion.

Nursing Diagnosis	Patient Outcomes	Nursing Interventions

LESSON 9 _____

Physical Assessment of Children

_____

🕮 **Reading Assignment:** Physical Assessment of Children (Chapter 10)
                            Standard Precautions (Appendix B)

Patients: Paul Parker, 24 months old, Well-Child Clinic, Room 202
               Sherrie Bedonie, 4 years old, Well-Child Clinic, Room 204
               Matthew Brown, 10 months old, Well-Child Clinic, Room 205
               Jason Baker, 14 years old, Pediatric Unit, Room 306

Assessment of children is important in order to gather information relating to their current health status. This lesson focuses on the steps of a thorough normal physical assessment for a 24-month-old boy, Paul Parker, who has come to the Well-Child Clinic for a checkup. Further opportunity for completion of charting for a physical assessment is provided when you visit 4-year-old Sherrie Bedonie, who has also come to the Well-Child Clinic. Opportunities exist for you to complete a comparison chart for both an infant's (Matthew Brown) and an adolescent's (Jason Baker) assessment, paying attention to developmental differences between these two children.

Objectives

Upon completion of this lesson, you will be able to:

1. Describe the steps in a physical assessment of a child.
2. Identify the findings of an assessment of a 24-month-old boy.
3. Chart findings from an assessment of a 4-year-old girl.
4. Compare physical assessments of an infant and an adolescent.

 Go to your textbook and read pp. 228-237 in Chapter 10, paying special attention to the steps of the health screening for a 2-year-old (pp. 229-231). Also, review Standard Precautions in Appendix B of your textbook (pp. 1062-1064).

1. Differentiate among the five basic ways that physical assessment data are gathered. Identify which of the senses (sight, hearing, smell, or touch) is used in each technique and describe their use.

Type	Senses Used	Description
Inspection		
Palpation		
Percussion		
Auscultation		
Smell		

2. Match each percussion sound with its description.

_____ Flat

_____ Dull

_____ Resonance

_____ Tympany

a. high-pitched loud sound heard over air-filled sections, such as the stomach

b. low-pitched sound from a hollow organ, such as the lungs

c. high-pitched soft sound over bone or muscle

d. medium-pitched sound over high-density organs, such as the liver

🖝 CD-ROM Activity

Walk through the lobby to the elevator and go to the Well-Child Clinic (Floor 2). Click on the **Nurses' Station** and sign in to see Paul Parker, a 24-month-old boy who has come with his mother for his 07:00 appointment in Room 202. Click Paul's **Patient Records** and review them. Write any important points that you have discovered in the space provided on the next page, making note of his normal assessment findings as well as those that are deviations from normal.

Student Notes—Paul's Chart

➤ Return to the Nurses' Station and click on **Physical Examination** and then on **Preliminary Examination**. Observe the nurse begin Jason's physical assessment by taking his measurements and temperature. (Remember to wash your hands before entering his room.)

3. Why are these anthropometrical measurements taken first?

4. List Paul's height, weight, head circumference, and temperature below.

Height

Weight

Head circumference

Temperature

➤ In questions 5 through 26, you will continue your assessment of Paul by clicking on each part of the Physical Examination and watching the nurse practitioner conduct each physical assessment. Refer to the corresponding sections in your textbook as you move through the assessment. Begin by clicking on the **Head & Neck** area of the 3-D model.

5. Where is Paul when the nurse performs his assessment, and what is her probable rationale for having him there?

In your textbook, refer to pp. 237-247 and Table 10-4 on p. 263.

Within the Head & Neck assessment, you are given three specific options. Click first on **EENT** and watch the ear, eye, nose, and throat assessment.

6. What area does the nurse practitioner examine first, and what is the rationale for this?

7. Record the findings of the assessment of Paul's scalp and hair.

8. For each category of the eye assessment listed below, give Paul's findings.

Category	Findings for Paul
Pupils	
Vision field	
Binocular vision	
External eye	

9. What are the findings of the assessment of Paul's ears?

10. What is the nurse practitioner inspecting when she looks in Paul's nose?

11. Assessment of the mouth shows second molars. Why is this important?

12. What does the visual examination of Paul's mouth show?

➤ Continue the Head & Neck assessment by clicking on **Lymphatics & Vascular** and then on **Cranial Nerves**. Observe these assessments.

13. What would be a positive sign during throat/neck palpation?

14. In the chart below and on the next page, briefly describe the way each cranial nerve can be assessed.

Cranial Nerve	How It Can Be Assessed
I—Olfactory Nerve	
II—Optic Nerve	

Cranial Nerve	How It Can Be Assessed
III—Oculomotor Nerve	
IV—Trochlear Nerve	
V—Trigeminal Nerve	
VI—Abducens Nerve	
VII—Facial Nerve	
VIII—Acoustic (Vestibulo-cochlear) Nerve	
IX—Glossopharyngeal Nerve	
X—Vagus Nerve	
XI—Spinal Accessory Nerve	
XII—Hypoglossal Nerve	

Read pp. 248-257 in your textbook.

Now click on the **Chest & Back** area of the 3-D model. View all sections of that assessment: Respiratory, Heart, and Musculoskeletal.

15. Describe the following types of breath sounds.

Rales

Rhonchi

Wheeze

16. Give the five steps in the heart auscultation process.

   a.

   b.

   c.

   d.

   e.

17. What is a heart murmur, and what does it sound like?

18. Summarize the findings of Paul's assessment in the areas listed below and on the next page.

Respiratory sounds

Heart sounds

Heart rate

Skin

→ Click on the **Abdomen** of the 3-D model and watch the assessment in the areas of Appearance, Bowel Sounds, and Pain & Masses.

19. Why are abdominal sounds auscultated in four different places?

20. What is assessed by palpating the abdomen?

📖 Read pp. 259-268 in your textbook.

→ Next, click on the **Upper Extremities** of the 3-D model. Observe the Vascular, Musculoskeletal, and Integumentary assessments. Then do the same for the **Lower Extremities**.

21. What were the findings regarding Paul's arms and legs?

22. List four different pulses that can be felt in the extremities.

    a.

    b.

    c.

    d.

→ Now click on the **Neurologic** assessment (the first button below the 3-D model).

23. Describe how tendon reflexes are checked.

24. Critique the nurse practitioner's assessment of Paul's reflexes.

→ Watch the assessment of Paul's **Gait**.

25. What is the purpose in having Paul pick up a toy?

Read pp. 257-259 in your textbook.

→ Return to the 3-D model and click on the **Genitalia** area. Observe the nurse practitioner's assessment.

26. Describe what the nurse practitioner would be looking for when screening for signs of sexual abuse?

→ Now that you have observed a physical assessment of a toddler, you find that you have the opportunity to watch a physical assessment of a 4-year-old girl. Return to the Nurses' Station and click on the **Login Computer**. Follow the onscreen instructions to sign out from working with Paul. Then sign in again, this time to see Sherrie Bedonie at 08:30. Click on her **Physical Examination** and on each separate assessment category, just as you did when watching Paul's assessment. (Wash your hands first!)

27. In the chart below and on the next page, summarize the assessment findings for Sherrie's complete examination as if you were doing the charting for the nurse practitioner.

Area	Charting for Sherrie
Preliminary Examination	
Head & Neck	
Chest & Back	
Abdomen	
Upper Extremities	
Lower Extremities	
Neurologic	

Area	Charting for Sherrie
Gait	
Genitalia	

28. Consider the assessments of Sherrie you just observed and compare them with those you watched for Paul. What changes were made in the mode of assessment, based on Sherrie's age?

You will now have the opportunity to compare physical assessments of an infant, 10-month-old Matthew Brown, and an adolescent, 14-year-old Jason Baker. To begin, go to the Nurses' Station and log out from seeing Sherrie by clicking on the **Supervisor's Computer**. Then log in to see Matthew Brown at 10:00, also in the Well-Child Clinic. Click on **Physical Examination** and observe each separate category of Matthew's assessment. As you watch, fill out his charting below and on the next page. When you have completed the charting, return to the Nurses' Station (wash your hands!) and log out from seeing Matthew on the Supervisor's Computer. Next, take the elevator to the Pediatric Unit (Floor 3). Once in that Nurses' Station, log in to see Jason Baker at 11:00 in Room 306. Complete Jason's portion of question 29 (below and on the next page) by reviewing his records (click on **Patient Records** and then on **Chart**) and by observing him post-operatively (click on **Patient Care**, then on **Data Collection**, and then on each area of the physical examination). Fill out Jason's charting as you proceed. (Remember to wash your hands before and after visiting him.) Finally, finish question 29 by describing the major differences in each of the listed categories between Matthew and Jason based on their ages and levels of physical maturity. If there is no developmental difference betweeen these patients in a category, record "ND."

29.

Area	Charting for Matthew	Charting for Jason	Developmental Differences
Preliminary Examination			
Head & Neck			

Area	Charting for Matthew	Charting for Jason	Developmental Differences
Chest & Back			
Abdomen			
Upper Extremities			
Lower Extremities			
Neurologic			
Gait			
Genitalia			

LESSON — **10** —————————————————————

Emergency Care of the Child

———

Reading Assignment: Emergency Care of the Child (Chapter 11)
Foundations of Child Health Nursing (Chapter 1)

Patient: Jason Baker, 14 years old, Pediatric Unit, Room 306

The need for emergency care of children is usually due to a sudden illness or injury. It is always a stressful time when a child must go to an emergency department. This lesson allows you to imagine yourself as the ED nurse providing the initial care for 14-year-old Jason Baker, who was brought to the hospital after fracturing his leg while playing basketball. You must anticipate the provision of care to both the injured teenager and his worried parents.

Objectives

Upon completion of this lesson, you will be able to:

1. Describe the first contact with an injured adolescent in the emergency department.
2. Conduct an emergency department interview.
3. Describe emergency department triage.
4. Obtain a health care consent for an injured teenager.
5. Describe a full emergency assessment of an injured adolescent.
6. Anticipate diagnostic testing for a child with a limb fracture.
7. Differentiate between an adult trauma scoring system and a pediatric trauma scoring system.
8. Assess an injured adolescent for shock.

Read pp. 272-276 in Chapter 11 in your textbook.

 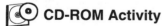 **CD-ROM Activity**

Take the elevator to the Pediatric Unit (Floor 3). Once in the Nurses' Station, log in to see Jason Baker at 05:30 (Room 306). Jason is a 14-year-old with a fractured leg. Observe the Case Overview and view your Assignment. Although you are on the Pediatric Unit, imagine yourself as the nurse with Jason in the emergency department when he first arrived by ambulance. Review Jason's history by clicking on **Patient Records** and then on his **Chart**. Inside his Chart, review the following sections: History & Physical, Nursing History, and Admissions Records. Use the space provided on the next page to write any notes of particular interest regarding Jason's emergency health needs when he first arrived in the emergency department.

Student Notes—Jason's Emergency Health Needs

Case Overview

History & Physical

Nursing History

Admissions Records

1. What is triage?

2. Describe the best ways for a nurse to communicate with an injured child in an emergency department.

3. If you were the nurse who first saw Jason in the emergency department, what would have been the first sentence you spoke to him?

4. Since Jason is 14 years old, how would you approach him to make your assessment?

5. Jason's traumatic injury is not uncommon in teenagers. Why?

6. Now that you have greeted Jason, what would you, as the ED nurse, do next?

 Read p. 16 in Chapter 1 of your textbook.

7. Who signed Jason's consent?

8. If the person you identified in question 7 had not been there, who would have been able to give consent for Jason?

Referring to pp. 276-281 and Tables 11-1 and 11-2 in Chapter 11 of your textbook, answer the following questions.

9. The parts of the primary emergency assessment are listed below. Next to each category, identify the type of data you would initially obtain from Jason if you were his ED nurse. Then list the findings from the ED History & Physical in Jason's Chart.

Assessment Categories	Data to Be Gathered	Findings from ED H&P
A = Airway Assessment		
B = Breathing		
C = Circulation		
D = Disability		
E = Expose		
F = Full Set of Vitals		
G = Give Comfort Measures		
H = Head-to-Toe Assessment		
I = Inspect Back and Isolate		

10. What other information would you gather regarding Jason's health? What were your findings about Jason in these areas?

11. What diagnostic tests do you anticipate would be needed for Jason? What tests were actually done on Jason, and what were the results?

Read pp. 285-289 in Chapter 11 of your textbook.

12. Based on the textbook's information specific to trauma, what changes would you make to your ED nursing assessment of Jason? List the questions to ask below.

13. What is a trauma score, and how does this score in children differ from that in adults?

14. How would you include Jason's mother and/or stepfather in his ED care?

15. Data in Jason's Case Overview reported that he also hit his head and was briefly unconscious. What further assessments would you make related to his neurologic status?

16. Based on Jason's vital signs in the ED History & Physical, did he come to the hospital in shock? Give a rationale for your answer.

The Child with a Chronic Condition or Terminal Illness

Reading Assignment: The Child with a Chronic Condition or Terminal Illness
  (Chapter 13)
  Foundations of Child Health Nursing (Chapter 1)
  Resources for Health Care Providers and Families (Appendix I)

Patients: De Olp, 6 years old, Pediatric Unit, Room 310
  Maria Ortiz, 8 years old, Pediatric Unit, Room 308

This lesson provides opportunities to anticipate the needs of chronically ill children and terminally ill children. You will be asked to consider nursing care for a child with a long-term health problem when you are introduced to Maria Ortiz, an 8-year-old with acute asthma, a chronic disease. After analyzing the effects of long-term health problems on Maria's growth and development, you will help her virtual brother and schoolmates understand her health needs. Then you will visit 6-year-old De Olp, who is receiving chemotherapy after being diagnosed with acute lymphocytic leukemia. Although acute lymphocytic leukemia is considered curable, this lesson moves forward in virtual time to events that, although remote, could occur in the future—metastasis resulting in a terminal diagnosis. The lesson concludes, therefore, with anticipatory nursing care for the dying De and her family. The ethical concerns of terminating treatment are also addressed.

Objectives

Upon completion of this lesson, you will be able to:

1. Differentiate between chronic and terminal disease.
2. Describe the effects of chronic and terminal illness on families.
3. Discuss how long-term health problems change growth and development in children.
4. Analyze Internet resources for families coping with chronic conditions.
5. Anticipate the reaction of siblings to chronic illness in a child.
6. Analyze concepts of dying in children.
7. Describe cultural influences related to dying.
8. Evaluate stages of dying.
9. Describe ethical considerations regarding ending treatment or life support.
10. Discuss hospice care.
11. Provide anticipatory guidance for palliative care.

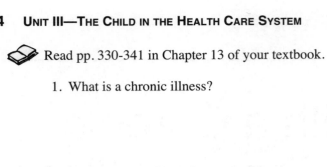 Read pp. 330-341 in Chapter 13 of your textbook.

1. What is a chronic illness?

2. Give eight examples of chronic health problems in children.

   a.

   b.

   c.

   d.

   e.

   f.

   g.

   h.

3. Why does a chronic illness become a situational crisis within a family?

4. How does the resilient family adjust to the situational crisis?

CD-ROM Activity

Take the elevator to the Pediatric Unit (Floor 3). Go to the Nurses' Station and log in to visit 8-year-old Maria Ortiz in Room 308 at 07:00. She is currently in respiratory distress due to an acute asthmatic episode. Click on **Patient Records** and then on her **Chart**. Read Maria's History & Physical, Nursing History, and Admissions Records. Use the space below to write down any pertinent points that pertain to chronic illness.

Student Notes—Maria's Chart

History & Physical

Nursing History

Admissions Records

5. How long has Maria had asthma?

6. What is Maria's perception of her illness?

7. A long-term illness such as asthma poses several problems relating to growth and development. For the nursing diagnosis listed below for Maria, identify two patient outcomes and nursing interventions to achieve those outcomes.

Nursing Diagnosis	Patient Outcomes	Nursing Interventions
Altered growth and development related to long-term condition		

8. What types of referrals or assistance will Maria need to ensure ongoing care at home?

9. What grade is Maria in at school? Describe a developmentally appropriate way to explain Maria's illness to her schoolmates.

10. Suppose, in this virtual world, that Maria had a 4-year-old brother. How might he react to her chronic illness?

11. How could the nurse help Maria's virtual brother cope with her long-term illness?

→ Return to the Nurses' Station and click **Leave the Floor**. Choose **Quit with Reset** to leave Canyon View Regional Medical Center. Then access the Internet using any web browser you wish.

Review the online community resources listed in Appendix I (pp. 1093-1100) in your textbook.

12. Find three websites of organizations that might provide information or support beneficial to Maria and her family. In the chart below, summarize what each organization could provide for Maria.

Organization	Website	Services Available
a.		
b.		
c.		

Return to your textbook and read pp. 342-352 in Chapter 13 and pp. 12-14 in Chapter 1.

➤ Return to Canyon View Regional Medical Center by restarting your *Virtual Clinical Excursions—Pediatrics* Patients' Disk. Go to Floor 3 and log in to see De Olp in Room 310 at 07:00. De has just been diagnosed with acute lymphocytic leukemia and is beginning chemotherapy treatments. Access her Chart and read her History & Physical, Nursing History, and Admissions Records. Write any pertinent points in the space below.

Student Notes—De's Chart

History & Physical

Nursing History

Admissions Records

➤ Acute lymphocytic leukemia is highly curable, and De is receiving a course of chemotherapy that is very likely to result in a complete cure. However, a small percentage of children with leukemia are not cured of their leukemia and subsequently die from the disease. Since you are caring for De in a virtual world, suppose that she has had two prior relapses of her leukemia and now has a metastasis to the brain, a common site of leukemic spread.

13. How old is De? Based on this, what would you anticipate her concept of death is?

14. According to the theorist Elisabeth Kübler-Ross, children go through the same stages of the dying process as adults. Below, list and describe how De might respond to each of the stages of dying.

Stage of Dying	De's Possible Response

15. De's parents would also have to cope with her death in this virtual world. How might they react to a terminal diagnosis?

16. How might De's grandparents react to a terminal diagnosis?

17. How can the nurse help De's family begin the grieving process?

18. Access De's Chart and review her Admissions Records regarding advance directives. If there were a signed advance directive in De's Chart, how would it be used?

19. Differentiate between palliative care and hospice care.

Palliative care

Hospice care

20. How might the following categories of care be undertaken if De were in hospice care for a leukemia-induced brain tumor metastasis?

Pain Control

Privacy

Family Routine

Nutrition

Responsiveness and Communication

Nursing Care of the Hospitalized Child

∽ **Reading Assignment:** The Ill Child in the Hospital and Other Settings (Chapter 12)
Principles and Procedures for Nursing Care of Children
(Chapter 14)
Medicating Infants and Children (Chapter 15)
Pain Management for Children (Chapter 16)
Standard Precautions (Appendix B)

Patients: Kaylie Sern, 3 years old, Pediatric Unit, Room 304
Maria Ortiz, 8 years old, Pediatric Unit, Room 308
Jason Baker, 14 years old, Pediatric Unit, Room 306

This lesson provides the opportunity to assess several hospitalized children of different ages. You will be able to visit each child and observe the interactions of the nurse with the child. Because these children are of different ages, the nurse's approach to each child's care should be different in the areas of safety, medication administration, intravenous therapy monitoring, oxygen therapy, assessment of pain, and preparing the child for surgery, including preoperative and postoperative nursing measures. The children include a toddler, a school-age child, and an adolescent. All are in the Pediatric Unit because of an acute illness or injury: Kaylie is dehydrated and has otitis media, Maria is suffering from asthma, and Jason, who has diabetes, fractured his leg and needs surgery.

Objectives

Upon completion of this lesson, you will be able to:

1. Describe developmental differences in children's reactions to illness and hospitalization.
2. Evaluate safety in the hospital.
3. Evaluate the measurement of children's vital signs.
4. Evaluate medication administration for children.
5. Evaluate IV monitoring for children.
6. Monitor oxygen delivery for a child.
7. Prepare children for procedures.
8. Describe preoperative and postoperative nursing interventions for children.
9. Analyze methods to identify and reduce pain in children.
10. Personalize a nursing care plan to reduce pain in an adolescent.

In your textbook read pp. 309-327 in Chapter 12 and pp. 421-426 in Chapter 16 on pain management in children.

1. For each age group listed below, describe the stressors associated with illness, hospitalization, and pain.

	Separation Anxiety	Fear of Injury or Pain	Loss of Control	Pain
Infant/toddler				
Preschool child				
School-age child				
Adolescent				

2. What are the three stages of separation anxiety in the infant and toddler? Describe the behavior that may accompany each stage.

a.

b.

c.

3. Discuss how parents and caretakers should be included in all aspects of a child's hospital stay.

💿 CD-ROM Activity

Go to the Pediatric Unit (Floor 3). At the Nurses' Station log in to visit Kaylie Sern in Room 304 at 07:00. Kaylie has been admitted to the hospital because she is severely dehydrated and has otitis media. Click on Kaylie's **Patient Records** and then her **Chart**. Review the Nursing History and Admissions Records. Once back in the Nurses' Station, review her Medication Administration Record (MAR), noting her medications for this morning. (Click on **Patient Records**, then on **MAR**.) Write any important points that you have discovered in the space provided below.

Student Notes—Kaylie's Chart and MAR

Nursing History

Admissions Records

MAR

4. Since Kaylie is 3 years old, how might she regress in her behavior as a result of her illness and hospitalization?

5. How can the nurse use the concept of therapeutic play to help Kaylie adjust to her illness and hospitalization?

 Return to your textbook and read pp. 356-364 in Chapter 14.

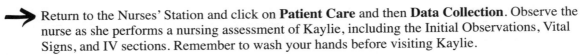 Return to the Nurses' Station and click on **Patient Care** and then **Data Collection**. Observe the nurse as she performs a nursing assessment of Kaylie, including the Initial Observations, Vital Signs, and IV sections. Remember to wash your hands before visiting Kaylie.

6. In evaluating the safety of the children under your care, what safety measures should you use when caring for Kaylie? What does the nurse in the video do to ensure Kaylie's safety?

7. In planning to care for Kaylie today, how would you approach morning care?

 Read pp. 364-370 in Chapter 14 of your textbook.

8. Taking vital signs on Kaylie is a challenge because of her age. Describe how you would do so.

9. Below, record Kaylie's vital signs values that were collected by the nurse and indicate whether they are normal (N) or abnormal (A).

10. Since Kaylie has a fever, efforts are made to reduce her fever. Name two nonpharmacologic methods of reducing fever.

Now turn to Chapter 15 in your textbook and read pp. 396-408.

11. What are the "six rights" to be checked before administering any medication?

   a.

   b.

   c.

   d.

   e.

   f.

→ You will now virtually jump ahead in time to view Kaylie's MAR at 09:00. In order to do so, you need to return to the Nurses' Station, click on the **Login Computer**, click on the **Supervisor's Computer** button, and then click the **Nurses' Station** button. Now reenter the Login Computer and sign in to see Kaylie at 09:00. Click on her **MAR** and review the medications she has received since 07:00.

12. What medication did Kaylie receive at 07:30? What is the procedure for giving that medication to a child?

Now review how to accurately compute drug calculations by referring to your pharmacology textbook or your nursing fundamentals textbook.

13. At 12:30 the nurse gave Kaylie pediatric acetaminophen elixir 225 mg PO. If the medication on hand was supplied as 80 mg per $\frac{1}{2}$ teaspoon, how many ml did the nurse give Kaylie?

14. How should the nurse measure the oral medication?

 Read the section on Intravenous Therapy on pp. 408-414 in Chapter 15 of your textbook. Also review Standard Precautions in Appendix B (pp. 1062-1064).

15. Kaylie has a running IV. Below, anticipate the infusion of the intravenous fluid by completing this chart for Tuesday between the hours of 07:00 and 11:00.

Time	Solution	Rate	Amount	Hourly Total	Site
07:00					
08:00					
09:00					
10:00					
11:00					

16. How did the nurse monitor Kaylie's IV status?

Return to the Nurses' Station and log out from seeing Kaylie by clicking on the **Supervisor's Computer** to reset the system. Then log in to visit Maria Ortiz at 09:00. Maria is an 8-year-old girl who is in the hospital because of an asthmatic episode. Click on her **Patient Records**, and then on her **Chart**. Read the Progress Notes and Physician Orders. Return to the Nurse's Station and review Maria's MAR and Kardex. Then visit Maria briefly by clicking on **Patient Care** and **Data Collection**. Observe the Initial Observations, Vital Signs, Chest & Back, and IV video sections. (Wash your hands!) Note important points relating to Maria's oxygen therapy, medications, and IV status in the space below.

Student Notes

Oxygen therapy

Respiratory treatments

Medications

IV status

17. What safety procedures and/or equipment-related aspects of health care should you plan to assess when you go to visit Maria?

 Read pp. 382-385 in Chapter 14 of your textbook.

18. Maria is getting oxygen via nasal cannula. What is the nurse's responsibility regarding the use of oxygen in the hospital setting?

19. The nurse tells you that she continues to find that Maria's nasal cannula has fallen off. What would you do if you were her nurse?

20. The nurse has asked you to get another pulse oximetry reading on Maria. What are the procedures to get this reading?

21. Maria has an IV running. How would your assessment of her IV status be similar to or different from the evaluation that you did of Kaylie's IV when you were with her?

22. Maria receives respiratory treatments. What is the nurse's responsibility during this therapy?

23. How can therapeutic play help Maria during her hospitalization?

Now return to your textbook and read on pp. 391-393 in Chapter 14.

→ You will now be visiting Jason Baker, a 14-year-old boy with diabetes who is scheduled for surgery to repair his leg fracture. Return to the Nurses' Station, click on the **Supervisors' Computer**, and log out from seeing Maria. Once back in the Nurses' Station, log in to visit Jason at 05:30 (Room 306). Access his Chart and review the Preoperative Instructions in the Operative Reports section. Then return to the Nurses' Station and review Jason's MAR. Note any important points in the space below.

Student Notes—Jason's Preoperative Needs

Operative Reports—Preoperative Instructions

MAR

→ Next, visit Jason in the Surgical Unit prior to his surgery. To do this, log out on the Supervisor's Computer. Then enter the open elevator and click button **4** to go to Surgery. Once in that unit's Nurses' Station, sign in to see Jason at 06:30. Participate in his nursing assessment by clicking on **Patient Care** and then **Data Collection**. View all assessments performed as part of Jason's pre-op care. (Remember to wash your hands before entering his room.)

24. What safety measures should be carried out when caring for Jason?

25. What patient preparation will you do for Jason prior to his surgery?

26. What parental preparation will you do for Jason's parents prior to his surgery?

27. Within the Operative Reports portion of Jason's Chart, review Jason's Preoperative Patient Instruction Sheet and Preoperative Checklist. Why is the completion of this checklist essential?

28. What is Jason wearing that must be removed before surgery? Why is this necessary?

29. How would you explain anesthesia to Jason?

30. Why did Jason receive cefazolin just before surgery? (*Hint:* To answer this question, look up the medication first in your own pharmacology book.)

→ Once again, jump ahead in virtual time to see Jason in the Post-Anesthesia Care Unit (PACU) after his surgery. To do this, log out on the Supervisor's Computer and take the elevator to Floor 4 (Surgery). Once there, log in to see Jason at 09:30 in the PACU. After listening to the Case Overview and Assignment, visit Jason in the PACU by clicking on **Patient Care** and **Data Collection**. (Wash your hands!) View all of the areas of this section.

31. What are the nursing actions that should be taken in the PACU (recovery room)?

32. Now that you have watched the nurse perform the assessment of Jason's leg, what did you see that was contrary to general nursing procedures?

33. How will the nurse know when Jason has adequately recovered from the anesthesia and he can return to the Pediatric Unit?

→ It is now time for Jason to return to the Pediatric Unit. Log out from the Surgical Unit by clicking on the **Supervisor's Computer**. Take the elevator to Floor 3 and log in to see Jason at 11:00. Click **Patient Care** and then **Data Collection**. Observe the nursing assessment, particularly the Initial Observations. Then return to the Nurses' Station and review the Physician Orders and Progress Notes in Jason's Chart. Finally, review his MAR. Below, record any information relating to his immediate postoperative needs.

Student Notes—Jason's Postoperative Needs

34. Now that Jason has returned to the Pediatric Unit from the PACU, what immediate nursing care should be given?

35. Why do Jason's postoperative orders indicate droperidol for nausea PRN? Write a summary of this medication below.

Return to your textbook and read pp. 426-435 in Chapter 16.

36. Describe two different methods of determining the presence of pain in children.

   a.

   b.

37. What criteria would the nurse use to determine whether to give Jason an IV analgesic or an oral analgesic?

Use a pharmacology textbook to review the analgesic medications that have been ordered for Jason.

38. Below, create medication cards for the drugs ordered for Jason. Include information on the action, side effects, and nursing implications of each medication.

Medication #1   **Medication #2**

Action

Side effects

Nursing implications

 39. Jason is to receive an IV push medication. After reviewing IV push administration in your textbook (pp. 412-413), describe the procedures the nurse used for giving Jason IV medications.

40. At 07:00 Tuesday, Jason received 3 mg IV of morphine sulfate. If the vial contained 5 mg in 2 ml, how many ml did the nurse give?

41. Besides medications, what other methods can the nurse use to reduce Jason's pain?

42. You suspect that Jason may be a candidate for patient-controlled analgesia (PCA). Prepare your remarks to advocate for PCA when you call the physician.

43. After reviewing the standardized nursing care plan for a child in pain on pp. 434-435 in Chapter 16 of your textbook, rewrite that care plan to personalize it for Jason's situation. Use resources available on your *Virtual Clinical Excursions—Pediatric* Patients' Disk to help. Click on **Planning Care**, then **Setting Priorities**, and then **Nursing Care Matrix**. Once you select the **Acute Pain** nursing diagnosis, click on **Outcomes & Interventions** to help you complete the table below. Remember to personalize the care plan for Jason by adding additional nursing outcomes and interventions.

Nursing Diagnosis	Patient Outcomes	Nursing Interventions
Acute pain related to being postoperative from bone fracture surgery		

LESSON **13**

The Child with a Fluid and Electrolyte Disorder

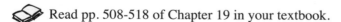

Reading Assignment: The Child with a Fluid and Electrolyte Alteration (Chapter 19)
NANDA-Approved Nursing Diagnoses 2001–2002
    Classification by Taxonomy II Domains (Appendix A)
Common Pediatric Laboratory Tests and Normal Values
    (Appendix H)

Patient: Kaylie Sern, 3 years old, Pediatric Unit, Room 304

This lesson focuses on the nursing care for Kaylie Sern, age 3 years, who is febrile and vomiting with severe dehydration. You will gather information on fluid and electrolyte imbalance in children. In addition, the questions in this lesson follow the nursing process from the assessment through evaluation components. You will also assess laboratory values, provide nursing measures, and prepare discharge teaching information for this ill child.

Objectives

Upon completion of this lesson, you will be able to:

1. Discuss fluid and electrolyte imbalance relating to dehydration in children.
2. Assess a child's hydration status.
3. Write the highest priority nursing diagnosis with the patient outcome.
4. Devise nursing interventions appropriate for rehydrating a toddler.
5. Develop interventions to help a child stop vomiting.
6. Evaluate the effectiveness of rehydration efforts.
7. Plan to provide health teaching of the parents prior to Kaylie's discharge home.

Read pp. 508-518 of Chapter 19 in your textbook.

CD-ROM Activity

Enter the lobby and take the elevator to the Pediatric Unit (Floor 3). Once there, go to the Nurses' Station and log in to visit Kaylie Sern in Room 304 at 07:00. Listen to your report on Kaylie (Case Overview and Assignment). Next, return to the Nurses' Station and click on **Patient Records** and then on **Chart**. Review the History & Physical, Nursing History, and the Admissions Records. Use the space below to write any important points that you have discovered regarding Kaylie's fluid and electrolyte status.

Student Notes—Kaylie's Chart

Case Overview

History & Physical

Nursing History

Admissions Records

1. Match each of the following terms with the correct definition.

    _____   Oliguria   a. Fluid within cells

    _____   Anuria   b. Fluid around cells

    _____   Intravascular fluid   c. Fluid in blood vessels

    _____   Interstitial fluid   d. Fluid between cells

    _____   Extracellular fluid   e. No urine output

    _____   Intracellular fluid   f. Scant urine output

2. What is dehydration?

3. In the table below, describe the different types of dehydration. Based on the data you have gathered, place an asterisk next to the type that best describes Kaylie's dehydration status.

Type of Dehydration	Description
Mild dehydration	
Moderate dehydration	
Severe dehydration	

4. List and describe nine nursing assessment findings that would indicate that Kaylie is severely dehydrated.

    a.

    b.

    c.

    d.

    e.

    f.

    g.

    h.

    i.

5. Below, record Kaylie's vital signs values taken in the Emergency Department (in her History & Physical). Identify whether each value is normal or abnormal and what that finding indicates.

Vital Signs at Admission	Value	Normal or Abnormal	Indication
Temperature			
Heart rate			
Respiratory rate			
Blood pressure			

→ Take a leap in virtual time to 09:00. To do this, log out on the Supervisor's Computer, return to the Nurses' Station, and log in again. This time sign in to see Kaylie at 09:00. Access Kaylie's EPR and review her Vital Signs summary. (Remember: Enter the password—nurse2b—and click on **Access Records**.)

6. Which of Kaylie's vital signs in question 5 are indicators that her body is not compensating for the fluid losses? Compare this to how her vital signs had changed by 07:15 (from her EPR). Describe why the changes occurred.

→ Return to the Nurses' Station, access Kaylie's Chart, and view her Laboratory Reports. (*Hint:* Review blood and urine laboratory tests and their normal and abnormal values. You can find this information in Appendix H, Common Pediatric Laboratory Tests and Normal Values, on pp. 1079-1092 in your textbook.)

7. List the values for the following lab tests drawn at 06:15. Indicate whether each is normal, high, or low.

Blood Chemistry Test	Value at 06:15	Normal, High, or Low
Hemoglobin		
Hematocrit		
Glucose		
Na^+		
K^+		
Cl^-		
CO_2		

8. On review of Kaylie's hematology results, why do her hemoglobin and hematocrit appear to be higher than normal?

9. Recalling Kaylie's blood glucose, describe what this value means.

10. What physiologic state is indicated by Kaylie's blood chemistries, including sodium (Na^+), potassium (K^+), chloride (Cl^-), and carbon dioxide (CO_2), along with her respiratory rate?
    a. Metabolic acidosis
    b. Metabolic alkalosis
    c. Respiratory acidosis
    d. Respiratory alkalosis

11. What is your rationale for your answer to question 10?

12. In the table below from your textbook, circle the phases of dehydration that are specific to Kaylie.

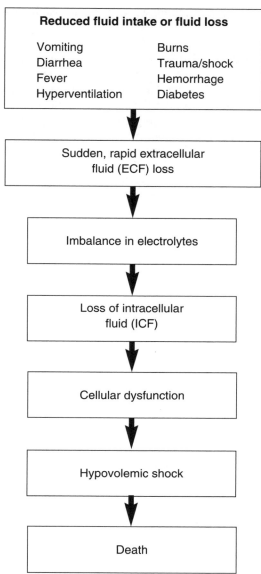

13. The specific gravity of Kaylie's urine output has been measured. What is a normal value for specific gravity? What is Kaylie's specific gravity value, and what does this indicate? Provide a rationale for your answer.

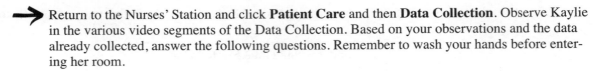 Return to the Nurses' Station and click **Patient Care** and then **Data Collection**. Observe Kaylie in the various video segments of the Data Collection. Based on your observations and the data already collected, answer the following questions. Remember to wash your hands before entering her room.

14. Based on the assessment findings, give the highest priority nursing diagnosis and the expected patient outcome for Kaylie. For help, click on **Planning Care**, **Setting Priorities**, and **Nursing Care Matrix**. Once you select the appropriate nursing diagnosis, click on **Outcomes & Interventions** to help you complete the table below. If you prefer, you can use the lists of NANDA Nursing Diagnoses in Appendix A of your textbook (pp. 1060-1061). Remember to personalize the care plan for Kaylie by adding additional nursing outcomes and interventions.

Nursing Diagnosis	Patient Outcomes	Nursing Interventions

15. How should the nurse provide fluids to Kaylie if she does not want to take them? (*Hint:* Remember that Kaylie is 3 years old.)

16. At 07:00, Kaylie's IV solution was changed from lactated Ringer's (LR) to D_5 .2NS @ 52 cc/hr. The IV bag contains 1000 cc. What time do you anticipate that the bag will need to be replaced? Complete your calculation in the space below.

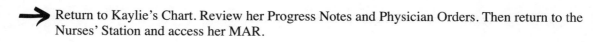 Return to Kaylie's Chart. Review her Progress Notes and Physician Orders. Then return to the Nurses' Station and access her MAR.

17. List the medications Kaylie is taking and explain how they might influence her hydration status.

18. Why are suppositories ordered instead of all oral medications?

 Return to your textbook and read pp. 524-527.

19. Kaylie's vomiting is also a factor in her dehydration. Discuss how effective the nursing interventions to alleviate her nausea were in each of the following areas.

   a. Antiemetic medications

   b. Oral intake

   c. Environmental stimuli

20. Why are neurologic checks ordered for Kaylie?

21. What are the findings from her neuro check performed at 07:15?

22. After Kaylie vomits, what nursing care measure would you offer her?

→ You will now jump ahead in virtual time to 13:00. In order to do this, return to the Nurses' Station, click on the **Supervisor's Computer**, and log off from this time period. Then log in again to see Kaylie at 13:00. Next, return to her EPR and review her Vital Signs and Intake & Output data.

23. In what way does Kaylie's temperature contribute to her dehydration at each of the following time periods?

Tuesday 06:00

Tuesday 09:00

24. Kaylie's first void in the hospital was 100 cc (at 10:00 hours). Find the output for her void at 13:00 hours on the I&O summary of the EPR. How does this latest output compare with a normal urine output for a toddler? (*Hint:* Use the formula on p. 516 of your textbook and show your calculation below.)

25. Below, list the types of intake and output that should be monitored when charting Kaylie's intake and output.

Types of Intake	Types of Outputs

26. What nursing measures, other than giving parenteral fluids, could help in the rehydration process since Kaylie continues to have some nausea?

27. What is Kaylie's diet order? When she is able to tolerate fluids, what additional fluid supplement can be used?

28. What topics should be included in the discharge teaching of Kaylie and her parents by the nurse?

The Child with Otitis Media

Reading Assignment: The Child with a Respiratory Alteration (Chapter 22)
The Child with a Sensory Alteration (Chapter 32)
NANDA-Approved Nursing Diagnoses 2001–2002
  Classification by Taxonomy II Domains (Appendix A)

Patients: Kaylie Sern, 3 years old, Pediatric Unit, Room 304
Paul Parker, 24 months old, Well-Child Clinic, Room 202

This lesson focuses on how two different children have been affected by otitis media, the most common ear infection in children. The nursing process is used to help you thoroughly assess the ears, devise nursing diagnoses, and plan and implement nursing care. The treatment of otitis media is discussed, and you will develop a teaching plan for parents who will be giving their child antibiotics for otitis media. You will have the opportunity to compare a child who had a surgical intervention to treat his otitis media with a child currently suffering from otitis media. Interventions will be evaluated, and revision for future care will be considered.

Objectives

Upon completion of this lesson, you will be able to:

1. Use the nursing process to care for children with otitis media.
2. Identify assessment criteria of the ear.
3. Conduct a nursing assessment of the ear.
4. Discuss antibiotic administration in children.
5. Develop a health teaching plan regarding otitis media.
6. Discuss reasons for tympanostomy tubes.
7. Describe how ear infections affect speech.

 First, review the textbook's coverage of the ear on pp. 1040-1041 in Chapter 32. Then read pp. 630-634 in Chapter 22.

1. What is otitis media?

2. Differentiate between two types of otitis media.

Type of Otitis Media	Description
Acute otitis media	
Otitis media with effusion	

3. List two causative microorganisms commonly linked to otitis media.

   a.

   b.

4. Discuss why children are more susceptible to otitis media than adults.

CD-ROM Activity

Take the elevator to the Pediatric Unit (Floor 3). Once in the Nurses' Station, log in to visit Kaylie Sern in Room 304 at 07:00. Listen to the Case Overview and Assignment. Below, write any important points regarding her ear infection.

Student Notes—Kaylie's Case Overview

→ Now, return to the Nurses' Station and click on **Patient Records** and then on **Chart**. Review the History & Physical, Nursing History, Progress Notes, and Physicians' Orders in Kaylie's Chart. Take notes below of any important points relating to her ear infection.

Student Notes—Kaylie's Chart

History & Physical

Nursing History

Progress Notes

Physicians' Orders

→ You will now visit Kaylie and her mother. Return to the Nurses' Station and click on **Patient Care** and then on **Data Collection**. Then click on the **Head & Neck** area of the 3-D body model and observe the assessment of the eyes, ears, nose, and throat (click on **EENT**). Keep notes below of any important points you discover. Remember to wash your hands before entering her room.

Student Notes—Assessment of Kaylie's Head & Neck

5. What physical assessment findings, if found, would indicate that Kaylie has a problem with her ears?

6. Toddlers have a limited ability to tell someone that they have pain. How could the nurse determine that Kaylie has ear pain?

7. Further assessment of Kaylie's ear infection is needed. What other assessments should the nurse be doing at this time? List these in the left column below. For each assessment you list, observe that segment of Kaylie's assessment and record the findings.

Assessments Needed   **Findings in Kaylie's Assessment**

8. Based on the nursing assessment of Kaylie's ear problems, list three nursing diagnoses in priority order that pertain to her health problem. Next to each diagnosis, write the expected short-term patient outcome. (*Hint:* You can refer to Appendix A on pp. 1060-1061 in your textbook for the list of NANDA diagnoses. Or you can return to the Nurses' Station, click on **Planning Care**, **Setting Priorities**, and **Nursing Care Matrix**. Once you select the appropriate nursing diagnosis, click on **Outcomes & Interventions** to help you complete the table below.)

Prioritized Nursing Diagnoses   **Short-Term Patient Outcome**

➤ Return to the Nurses' Station and review Kaylie's Medication Administration Record by clicking on **Patient Records** and then on **MAR**.

9. At 08:30, what medication did the nurse administer? What should the nurse have done before this medication was given?

10. Since Kaylie will be on a course of amoxicillin to treat her otitis media, develop a health teaching plan to advise her parents how to go about this treatment.

➤ You have learned that a child with a history of otitis media is being seen in the Well-Child Clinic today. Go to the Nurses' Station and log out of the Pediatric Unit on the Supervisor's Computer. Then take the elevator to Floor 2. At the Well-Child Clinic Nurses' Station, log in to see Paul Parker, age 24 months, in Room 202 at 07:00.

After listening to the Course Overview, return to the Nurses' Station and click on **Physical Examination**. (Remember to wash your hands.) Once inside the room, click on the **Head & Neck** area of the 3-D model. Then click on **EENT** and observe the eye, ear, nose, and throat assessment performed by the nurse practitioner. Jot down any important notes below.

Student Notes—Paul's Head & Neck Assessment

11. List the parts of the Head & Neck assessment that are pertinent for a child with a history of otitis media.

12. During Paul's assessment, what does the nurse practitioner see in his ears?

→ Return to the Nurses' Station and click on **Patient Records**. Inside Paul's Chart, review the Well-Child Visits, Sick-Child Visits, and Referral Forms.

13. What are PET tubes, and why are they used?

14. For each of Paul's episodes of ear infection (listed by age below), identify what measures were taken to treat his otitis media.

Age of Otitis Media Episode	Treatment Used
6 months	
7 months	
9 months	
10 months	
12 months	
14 months	

15. Discuss why the administered antibiotics changed for each of Paul's episodes of otitis media.

16. The nurse practitioner earlier assessed Paul's hearing. Check his Chart again for the most current Hearing & Vision Screening. Discuss the findings of Paul's hearing test.

17. Paul's mother is concerned about his speech since he has had so many ear infections. Provide information on any referrals written for Paul for speech evaluation.

18. How would ear infections affect Paul's speech?

19. In each of the following categories, what comparisons can be made between Kaylie's and Paul's health needs regarding their otitis media?

Category	Kaylie	Paul
Medications		
History of otitis media		
Hearing screening		
Speech		

LESSON 15

The Child with Asthma

Reading Assignment: The Child with a Respiratory Alteration (Chapter 22)
Principles and Procedures for Nursing Care of Children
  (Chapter 14)
NANDA-Approved Nursing Diagnoses 2001–2002
  Classification by Taxonomy II Domains (Appendix A)
Resources for Health Care Providers and Families (Appendix I)

Patient: Maria Ortiz, 8 years old, Pediatric Unit, Room 308

Providing nursing care to a child experiencing an acute asthmatic episode is the focus of this lesson. You will care for Maria Ortiz, an 8-year-old who experiences increasing levels of respiratory compromise. During the lesson, you will assess Maria's visit to the emergency department, as well as her nursing needs after she is admitted to the Pediatric Unit. In addition, you will be required to identify a sudden change in her health and take action immediately.

Objectives

Upon completion of this lesson, you will be able to:

1. Describe asthma.
2. Differentiate among breath sounds in asthma.
3. Identify factors making a child at risk for asthma.
4. Assess respiratory status in a child with asthma.
5. Recognize the need for further nursing care for a child with asthma.
6. Personalize a standardized care plan for a child hospitalized with asthma.

Refresh your knowledge about the respiratory system by reading pp. 622-626 in Chapter 22 of your textbook.

1. Match each of the following terms with its correct definition or description.

_____ Hypercapnia

_____ Hypoxia

_____ Nasal flaring

_____ Stridor

_____ Retractions

_____ Orthopnea

_____ Tachypnea

a. Rapid respiratory rate

b. Harsh, shrill sound indicating constriction of airway

c. Difficulty with breathing unless upright

d. Decreased O_2 in tissues

e. Increased CO_2 in blood

f. Using accessory chest muscles to breath

g. Needing to use widening of nares to take in more air

Read pp. 661-672 in Chapter 22 of your textbook.

2. What are the three presumptive signs of asthma?

a.

b.

c.

3. List six risk factors for the development of asthma in children.

a.

b.

c.

d.

e.

f.

4. How do allergens play a role in the development of asthma?

5. Describe pulmonary function testing.

6. Differentiate among rales, rhonchi, and wheezing.

Rales

Rhonchi

Wheezing

 Read pp. 384-385 in Chapter 14 of your textbook.

7. What is a pulse oximetry reading?

8. What is a normal pulse oximetry reading ($SpO_2\%$) for children?

9. How should a pulse oximetry reading be obtained on a child?

CD-ROM Activity

Take the elevator to the Pediatric Unit (Floor 3). Once in the Nurses' Station, log in to visit Maria Ortiz, age 8 years, who is in Room 308. The time is 07:00. Listen to the Case Overview and read the Assignment on Maria. Write any important points in the space below.

Case Overview and Assignment—Maria Ortiz

Next, return to the Nurses' Station, access Maria's Patient Records, and open her Chart. Review the History & Physical section of the Chart, focusing on the Emergency Department History and Physical. Also review Maria's Nursing History, Admissions Records, Physician Orders, and Progress Notes. Record any important points regarding her asthma in the space provided below.

Student Notes

History & Physical

Nursing History

Admissions Records

Physician Orders

Progress Notes

10. Based on your review of Maria's Emergency Department History and Physical, what information has been gathered regarding the presumptive cause of Maria's current asthmatic episode?

11. If you had conducted the emergency department intake for Maria, what other information would you have gathered?

→ Return to the Nurses' Station and click on **Patient Care** and then on **Data Collection**. View the Initial Observations, Vital Signs, and Chest & Back assessments. Remember to wash your hands before entering her room.

12. Based on your observation of Maria in her room, what nursing assessment findings indicate that she is in respiratory distress?

13. Are Maria's breath sounds indicative of asthma? Provide a rationale for your answer.

14. Compare Maria's respiratory status with the usual clinical picture of a child with asthma.

Return to the Nurses' Station and access Maria's MAR. You can find it by clicking on **Patient Records** and then on **MAR**, or you can simply click on the MAR notebook on the counter inside the Nurses' Station.

In your pharmacology book, review the medications listed in Maria's MAR.

15. In the chart below, identify the type, action, side effects, and nursing implications of each of Maria's medications.

Medication	Type	Action	Side Effects	Nursing Implications
Solu-medrol 30 mg IV q6h				
Albuterol nebulizer				

Now jump ahead in virtual time to 11:00. To do this, return to the Nurses' Station and click on the Login Computer and then on the **Supervisor's Computer** button. Next, return to the Nurses' Station and sign in to work with Maria at 11:00. Access her latest Patient Records and read the Progress Notes in her Chart. Next, review her EPR. Enter the password—nurse2b—and click on **Access Records**. Within the EPR, assess Maria's vital signs, including her pulse oximetry readings.

16. Below list Maria's SpO_2% from 08:30 through 11:00. What does this trend show?

Time	SpO_2%	Trend
08:30		
09:00		
09:30		
10:00		
10:30		
11:00		

17. When Maria's oxygen saturation dropped at 10:30 to 89%, why did she become anxious?

18. Because Maria obviously has a compromised airway, what should the nurse do first?

→ Return to the Nurses' Station and listen to Maria talking at 11:00 by clicking on **Patient Care** and **Data Collection**. Observe the videos for Vital Signs, Head & Neck, and Behavior.

19. What is your assessment of Maria's speech pattern at this time? What does her speech pattern suggest to you about her respiratory status? What is the correct term for this?

20. Since Maria is having difficulty keeping her nasal cannula in place, what would you recommend?

→ Make another jump forward in virtual time to 13:00 by using the same procedure as before. Keep Maria as your patient, but switch to the 13:00–14:29 period of care. Again, visit Maria in her room again and observe the assessments of her Vital Signs, Head & Neck, Chest & Back, and Behavior. Then return to the Nurses' Station and review her MAR. Finally, read the Progress Notes in her Chart.

21. How has Maria's respiratory status been since 11:00? Provide a rationale for your answer.

22. Check Maria's STAT medication orders in her MAR for 11:00. How did the albuterol treatment and the IV bolus of methylprednisolone sodium affect Maria's respiratory status?

23. What is status asthmaticus?

24. What signs would indicate that Maria was developing status asthmaticus?

25. What would you say to Maria's mother if she stated, "Isn't asthma due to being high strung? It's shameful that Maria gets upset and gets asthma."

→ Now that Maria is stabilized, conduct a more through psychosocial interview by asking her about the effects of asthma on her life. From the Nurses' Station, click on **Patient Care** and **Data Collection**. Then, once inside her room, click on **Behavior**. Record your findings in question 26.

26. Based on your assessment of Maria's behavior, describe the effects asthma has had on the following areas of her life.

Schoolwork

Exercise

Nutrition and diet

27. Differentiate between the use of a nebulizer and a metered-dose inhaler.

Nebulizer

Metered-dose inhaler

28. Why might Maria be given a peak flowmeter to use after discharge?

Analyze the nursing care plan for The Child Hospitalized with Asthma on pp. 667-670 in your textbook.

Personalize the textbook's standardized care plan for Maria. Use the resources on your *Virtual Clinical Excursions—Pediatrics* Patients' Disk to help you do this. Click on **Planning Care**, **Setting Priorities**, and **Nursing Care Matrix**. Once you select the appropriate nursing diagnosis, click on **Outcomes & Interventions** to help you complete the table in question 29. (Or you can use the lists of NANDA Nursing Diagnoses in Appendix A on pp. 1060-1061 of your textbook.)

29. Below and on the next page, personalize the care plan for Maria by providing additional nursing outcomes and interventions for each diagnosis you identify,

Nursing Diagnosis	Patient Outcomes	Nursing Interventions

a.

b.

Nursing Diagnosis	Patient Outcomes	Nursing Interventions
c.		
d.		

 Maria's mother says that she likes to get health information from the Internet. You decide to pre-screen some appropriate websites for her regarding asthma. Sign on to the web browser of your choice and visit some of the websites listed in Appendix I (Resources for Health Care Providers and Families) beginning on p. 1093 of your textbook.

30. Below, summarize the usefulness of each website you visited.

Organization	Website	Services Available
a.		
b.		
c.		

Note: Discharge planning and health teaching for Maria is included in Lesson 20.

LESSON 16

The Child with Leukemia

∽ Reading Assignment: The Child with Cancer (Chapter 25)

The Child with a Neurologic Alteration (Chapter 29)

NANDA-Approved Nursing Diagnoses 2001–2002
   Classification by Taxonomy II Domains (Appendix A)

Resources for Health Care Providers and Families (Appendix I)

Patient: De Olp, 6 years old, Pediatric Unit, Room 310

In this lesson you will provide nursing care to 6-year-old De Olp, who was diagnosed with acute lymphocytic leukemia 4 days ago. You will review all aspects of leukemia in children, review the health care De has received since her diagnosis, and then care for her in the pediatric setting. De has had invasive cancer diagnostic testing and is currently undergoing chemotherapy treatments.

Objectives

Upon completion of this lesson, you will be able to:

1. Describe cancer and, specifically, acute lymphocytic leukemia.
2. Differentiate among various diagnostic tests and their findings for children who have acute lymphocytic leukemia.
3. Discuss the chemotherapeutic medications prescribed for De.
4. Develop a nursing care plan designed to focus on alleviation of side effects produced by specified antineoplastic agents.
5. Follow a child's course of intrathecal and intravenous chemotherapy.
6. Provide monitoring of vital signs for a child with acute lymphocytic leukemia.
7. Personalize a nursing care plan for a child with acute lymphocytic leukemia.
8. Intervene when a child's health condition changes.
9. Provide support to the family of a child with leukemia.
10. Analyze Internet resources for families coping with a child who has cancer.

Read pp. 774-781 in Chapter 25 of your textbook.

1. Match each of the following terms relating to cancer with its correct definition.

   _____ Metastasis   a. Extent of disease

   _____ Carcinogen   b. Cell growth at site of origin

   _____ Invasion   c. Cells spreading to distant areas

   _____ Tumor staging   d. Causation

2. What are the seven cardinal signs of cancer in children?

   a.

   b.

   c.

   d.

   e.

   f.

   g.

Return to your textbook and read pp. 781-790.

3. What is acute lymphocytic leukemia (ALL)?

4. How is the bone marrow implicated in the course of leukemic disease?

5. Why is the triad of anemia, thrombocytopenia, and leukocytosis so important in leukemia? Define each of these terms.

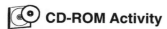 **CD-ROM Activity**

Go to the Nurses' Station on Floor 3 (Pediatric Unit). Once there, sign in for a 07:00 visit to De Olp, age 6 years, in Room 310. In order to care for De today, you must review her history since her admission on Saturday. Click on **Patient Records** and then on **Chart**. Read De's History & Physical, the Nursing History, Admissions Records, Physician Orders, Progress Notes, Laboratory Reports, and Operative Reports. Below and on the next page, record any pertinent points pertaining to her leukemia between Saturday and this morning.

Student Notes

History & Physical

Nursing History

Admissions Records

Physician Orders

Progress Notes

Laboratory Reports

Operative Reports

6. List the presenting signs from De's Saturday History & Physical that were a direct result of the leukemic triad.

7. Why was blood typing ordered for De?

8. Below, list De's laboratory results on admission. What do they mean? (*Hint:* See Appendix H, Common Pediatric Laboratory Tests and Normal Values on pp. 1079-1092 of your textbook to help you interpret the results.)

Blood Test	Results on Admission	Meaning of Results
White blood cells		
Hemoglobin		
Hematocrit		
Platelets		

9. How would you answer De's father when he asks, "How did she get leukemia?"

10. Review the results of De's urinalysis obtained on Saturday. What did this urinalysis indicate?

11. On Saturday, what were De's PT, INR, and PTT values? What did this indicate?

12. What is a biopsy procedure?

13. Why did De have a bone marrow aspiration and biopsy?

14. If you were the health care professional who had to explain the bone marrow aspiration procedure to De and her father, what would you say?

15. After the bone marrow aspiration, De had a lumbar puncture. Why was that procedure done?

Review the textbook discussion of bone marrow aspiration on p. 775 in Chapter 25 and lumbar puncture on pp. 945-946 in Chapter 29.

16. What immediate nursing care, other than taking vital signs, is important to implement for De after each of the following diagnostic tests were undertaken?

Bone marrow aspiration and biopsy

Lumbar puncture

17. Review De's bone marrow aspiration and biopsy reports in her chart. Explain how the findings indicate acute lymphocytic leukemia.

18. De had a right subclavian vein single lumen port-a-cath placed for chemotherapy on Monday. What is the advantage of having this catheter placed rather than a peripheral IV?

→ Return to De's Chart and review the Informed Consent for the Administration of Cancer Chemotherapy that her father signed (the last page in the Admissions Records section). Then review the Medication Records in her Chart.

19. Why is the signed informed consent important? (Give at least two different reasons.)

   a.

   b.

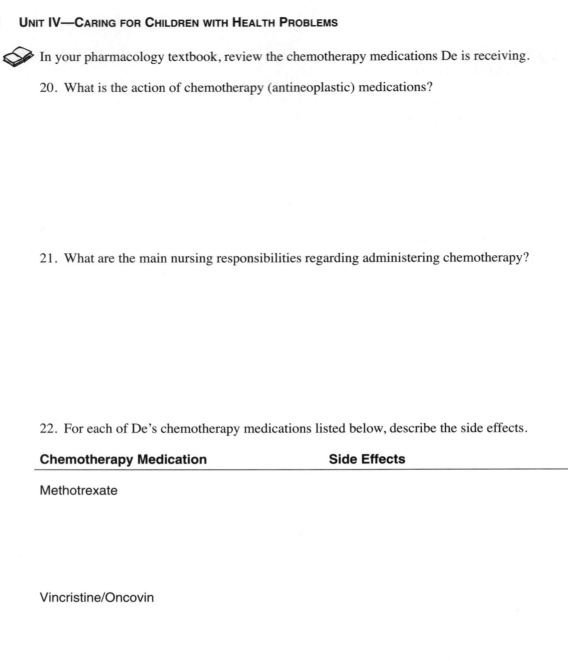 In your pharmacology textbook, review the chemotherapy medications De is receiving.

20. What is the action of chemotherapy (antineoplastic) medications?

21. What are the main nursing responsibilities regarding administering chemotherapy?

22. For each of De's chemotherapy medications listed below, describe the side effects.

Chemotherapy Medication	Side Effects
Methotrexate	
Vincristine/Oncovin	
Asparanginase/ Elspar	

23. When will the side effects of chemotherapy most likely begin to appear in De's case?

24. Below, devise a nursing care plan for De, focusing on preventing and/or minimizing the side effects of the chemotherapeutic medications she is receiving. The list of nursing diagnoses is in Appendix A (pp. 1060-1061) of your textbook.

Nursing Diagnosis	Patient Outcomes	Nursing Interventions

25. Why did De receive several chemotherapy drugs at the same time?

26. Before treatment can begin, De must be treated for her abnormal electrolyte levels. What in her Chart indicates these abnormal levels? How is this being treated? Why?

27. The first stage of chemotherapy treatment for De's ALL includes induction. What does this mean?

28. How is an intrathecal medication given?

29. Why did De receive her methotrexate intrathecally?

Return to your pharmacology textbook to review more about De's other medications.

30. What is allopurinol, and why is De receiving it?

31. De is also on dexamethasone (Decadrol). Why were these drugs prescribed for her?

If you did not listen to De's Case Overview and read the Assignment, do so now. Return to the Nurses' Station and click on **Patient Care**, **Case Overview**, and **Assignment**. Then click on **Patient Records** and review her Kardex. Make note of anything you need to know about De below.

Case Overview and Assignment

Kardex

32. Now that you have familiarized yourself with De Olp's health needs, what are your nursing goals for today (Tuesday) for the time you will spend caring for De?

→ Now go to De's room to take her vital signs. You can do this by clicking **Patient Care** and **Data Collection**. Wash your hands before entering the patient's room. Inside De's room, click on **Vital Signs**.

33. Below, list De's vital signs for Tuesday at 07:00 and indicate whether each value is normal (N) or abnormal (A).

34. What is the most important short-term patient outcome for this time that you will spend with De?

35. How will you do that?

→ Continue your nursing assessment of De by clicking on other sections of the Data Collection.

36. What is the status of De's port-a-cath?

37. Describe De's bone marrow aspiration site.

➤ It is now time to jump in virtual time to 11:00. You can do this by returning to the Nurses' Station and clicking on the Supervisor's Computer. Next, return to the Nurses' Station and sign in to work with De at 11:00. Click **Patient Care** and **Data Collection** and fully assess De again.

38. By 11:00 you notice changes in De's respiratory status. What are these changes?

39. What is your next nursing action?

➤ Once again, jump ahead in virtual time, now to 13:00. Once there, listen to the Case Overview. Then review De's Chart and MAR.

40. What is the drug furosemide, and why did De receive it today?

41. What nursing care should be given to De after she receives the furosemide?

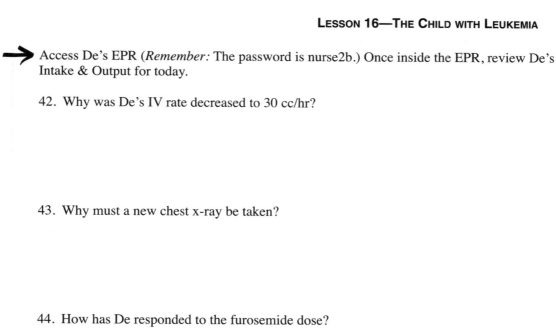

Access De's EPR (*Remember:* The password is nurse2b.) Once inside the EPR, review De's Intake & Output for today.

42. Why was De's IV rate decreased to 30 cc/hr?

43. Why must a new chest x-ray be taken?

44. How has De responded to the furosemide dose?

45. How can the nurse encourage De's father to be a part of her hospital care?

Review the nursing care plan printed in your textbook on pp. 783-789. Your next task is to personalize the textbook's care plan for De. To do this, you can click on **Planning Care**, **Setting Priorities**, and **Nursing Care Matrix**. Once you select the appropriate nursing diagnosis, click on **Outcomes & Interventions** to help you complete question 46. If you prefer, you can use the lists of NANDA Nursing Diagnoses in Appendix A of your textbook (pp. 1060-1061).

46. Below and on the next page, create a personalized care plan for De.

Nursing Diagnosis	Patient Outcomes	Nursing Interventions
a.		

b.

c.

d.

e.

47. What should be the recommendations regarding vaccinations for De?

48. De's father stops you as you say goodbye at the end of your period of care. "Thank you for taking care of my De today," he says. "Since you're a student nurse, I bet you're up on the latest treatments for things. Do you think De would need a bone marrow transplant or something like that?" How do you answer his question? What is he really asking you?

 Review the online community resources for families with children with cancer listed in Appendix I (Resources for Health Care Providers and Families) on pp. 1093-1100 of your textbook.

49. Select three websites of organizations that would be of help to De and her father, considering her health needs. Visit these websites using the browser of your choice and write a summary of what is available online relating to children with leukemia.

Organization	Website	Services Available

The Child with a Leg Fracture

/OⱭ **Reading Assignment:** The Child with a Musculoskeletal Alteration (Chapter 27)
NANDA-Approved Nursing Diagnoses 2001–2002
Classification by Taxonomy II Domains (Appendix A)

Patient: Jason Baker, 14 years, Pediatric Unit, Room 306

In this lesson, you are given the opportunity to provide nursing care to Jason Baker, age 14 years, who suffered a fractured tibia-fibula. Jason's hospitalization has included a surgical procedure for open reduction of his fractures. Therefore, you will be able to monitor his leg postoperatively. This includes caring for a fresh cast and assessing for prevention of complications in a casted limb. Discharge planning regarding cast care is also included. (Please refer to Lesson 12 regarding the preoperative care of Jason and alleviation of pain postoperatively.)

Objectives

Upon completion of this lesson, you will be able to:

1. Review the emergency department's evaluation of an adolescent with a fractured leg.
2. Discuss nursing care of an adolescent with a fracture.
3. Assess cast care.
4. Develop nursing care plans to reduce the risk for postprocedural complications relating to cast care.
5. Develop a discharge planning summary relating to home care of a cast.
6. Discuss use of traction.

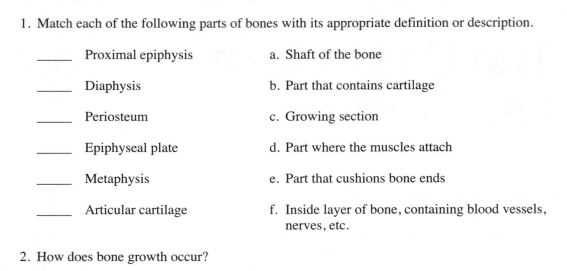 In your textbook, read pp. 852-856, 859-861, and 874-878 in Chapter 27.

1. Match each of the following parts of bones with its appropriate definition or description.

_____ Proximal epiphysis   a. Shaft of the bone

_____ Diaphysis   b. Part that contains cartilage

_____ Periosteum   c. Growing section

_____ Epiphyseal plate   d. Part where the muscles attach

_____ Metaphysis   e. Part that cushions bone ends

_____ Articular cartilage   f. Inside layer of bone, containing blood vessels,
                                        nerves, etc.

2. How does bone growth occur?

3. Where does the growth of long bones occur?

4. How does a bone fracture heal?

CD-ROM Activity

Take the elevator to the Pediatric Unit (Floor 3). Go to the Nurses' Station and log in to see Jason Baker in Room 306 at 05:30. Jason is a 14-year-old boy who was admitted yesterday after fracturing his leg during a basketball game. Watch the Case Overview and click on **Assignment** to get a report. Then return to the Nurses' Station and click on **Patient Records** and **Chart**. Inside the Chart, read Jason's History & Physical, Nursing History, Admissions Records, and Physician Orders regarding his medications. Limit your data gathering to information regarding his leg fracture. Write down important points below.

Student Notes—Jason Baker

Case Overview and Assignment

History & Physical

Nursing History

Admission Records

Physician Orders—Medications

5. In this virtual world, if you had been at the basketball game when Jason fell, what nursing assessment findings would have led you to suspect a leg fracture?

6. If you had been the nurse gathering data from Jason in the emergency department, what additional information would you have gathered?

→ Now click on **X-Rays & Diagnostics** (still inside Jason's Chart) and review his x-ray findings. Write down any important information below.

X-ray results

7. Describe the difference between a simple fracture and a compound fracture. Put an asterisk next to the type of fracture that Jason has.

Simple

Compound

8. What color would Jason's leg be on the x-ray film?

➡ Read Jason's Operative Reports in his Chart.

9. How would you explain the procedures to Jason, his mother, and his stepfather?

10. Identify two types of casts and describe their strengths and weaknesses.

Type of Cast	Strengths	Weaknesses

11. List the layers of a completed cast from skin-side to outside.

a.

b.

c.

➡ Jason has gone to surgery and is now in the Post-Anesthesia Care Unit (PACU). In order to go there to care for him, you need to log out first. Return to Nurses' Station and sign out on the Supervisor's Computer. Then return to the Nurses' Station and take the elevator to Floor 4 (Surgery). Once there, log in to see Jason at 09:30. Listen to the Case Overview and read the Assignment. Next, click on **Patient Care** and observe the Data Collection done in the PACU. Focus on the postoperative assessments done by the nurse. You can do this by clicking on **Initial Observations**, **Lower Extremities**, and **Wound Condition**, as well as other areas of the assessment. Remember to wash your hands before entering his room.

12. What kind of cast does Jason have? What nursing care must be given to Jason while his cast dries?

13. List and describe five nursing assessments to be made relating to cast care.

    a.

    b.

    c.

    d.

    e.

14. Why must the observations listed in question 13 be made?

15. Based on your observation of the nurse's assessment of Jason's leg, what is wrong about the nurse's assessment skills?

→ Jason has now been transferred back to the Pediatric Unit. Again, log out on the Supervisor's Computer and take the elevator back to Floor 3 (Pediatric Unit). Once there, sign in to do a nursing assessment of Jason at 11:00. Click on **Patient Care** and **Data Collection** and observe all sections of the physical assessment.

16. Enter your assessment findings for Jason below.

Vital signs

Lower extremities

Cast

17. When should your next nursing assessment be? Why?

18. What would indicate that Jason was bleeding inside his cast?

19. Why is Jason's casted leg on pillows?

20. Since Jason's leg may have some swelling over the next 24 to 48 hours, what can the nurse do to minimize this possibility?

21. If Jason's incisions were infected under his cast, how would you know?

22. What are the negative effects of immobility for a child with a cast?

23. Below and on the next page, write a nursing care plan including two nursing diagnoses for Jason related to the hazards of immobility while he is recuperating from his surgery. Refer to Appendix A of your textbook for the list of NANDA nursing diagnoses (pp. 1060-1061).

Nursing Diagnosis	Patient Outcomes	Nursing Interventions

Nursing Diagnosis	Patient Outcomes	Nursing Interventions

24. What additional consults should be ordered for Jason related to his decreased mobility?

25. Jason's nursing care must include assessment for the complication of fat emboli. For the nursing diagnosis below, write the Patient Outcome and Nursing Interventions specifically for Jason's nursing care.

Nursing Diagnosis	Patient Outcome	Nursing Interventions
Risk for Injury: Fat Emboli related to fracture of a long bone		

26. Development of compartment syndrome is a serious potential complication of limb fractures. For the nursing diagnosis below, write the Patient Outcome and Nursing Interventions specifically for Jason's nursing care.

Nursing Diagnosis	Patient Outcomes	Nursing Interventions
Risk for Ineffective Tissue Perfusion: Peripheral related to casted limb		

27. Develop a discharge teaching tool to give to Jason and his parents regarding care of his cast at home.

28. Jason's stepfather asks you how Jason's leg fracture might affect him since he is still growing. How will you respond?

29. Considering Jason's developmental level, what fears may Jason have regarding going home with a cast?

➤ Return to the Nurses' Station and click on **Patient Records** and **Chart**. Read the Physician Orders regarding Jason's ambulation.

30. What are the physician orders for Jason's ambulation and physical therapy?

31. Using the nursing diagnosis below, develop a nursing care plan to serve as the basis for health teaching for Jason based on his ambulation orders.

Nursing Diagnosis	Patient Outcomes	Nursing Interventions
Risk for Falls related to crutch walking		

 Return to your textbook and read pp. 856-859 in Chapter 27.

32. One of Jason's visitors asks you why Jason isn't in traction. What is your answer?

33. If Jason asks you how the cast will be removed once his leg heals, how will you answer him?

34. What skin care will you teach Jason and his parents to do after the cast is removed?

The Child with Diabetes Mellitus

∽ **Reading Assignment:** Caring for the Child with an Endocrine or Metabolic Alteration
(Chapter 28)
NANDA-Approved Nursing Diagnoses 2001–2002
Classification by Taxonomy II Domains (Appendix A)
Resources for Health Care Providers and Families (Appendix I)

Patient: Jason Baker, 14 years, Pediatric Unit, Room 306

Providing nursing care to an adolescent with type 1 diabetes mellitus (DM) is the focus of this lesson. You will again care for Jason Baker, this time focusing on his history of having diabetes mellitus. As a 14-year-old, Jason needs additional care since his diabetes affects the healing process for his fractured leg. Therefore, you will spend time learning the pathophysiology of diabetes mellitus, the signs of DM in children, treatment modalities, nursing care, and patient education needs for Jason and his family.

Objectives

Upon completion of this lesson, you will be able to:

1. Discuss the physiologic mechanism behind diabetes mellitus.
2. Discuss the use of different insulins and apply this knowledge to an adolescent's care.
3. Analyze diet modifications for an adolescent with diabetes mellitus.
4. Prepare a presentation comparing hypoglycemia and hyperglycemia.
5. Develop a health teaching brochure on complications of diabetes mellitus.
6. Personalize a nursing care plan for an adolescent with type 1 diabetes mellitus.
7. Discuss the developmental effects of diabetes mellitus on an adolescent.
8. Search for websites designed to help children and families learn more about diabetes mellitus.

Read pp. 922-938 in Chapter 28 of your textbook.

1. Differentiate between type 1 and type 2 diabetes mellitus.

Type 1 DM

Type 2 DM

2. Describe the incidence of type 1 and type 2 DM in children today.

3. Describe the physiologic mechanism behind the interaction between insulin and glucose in the body.

4. How does the absence of insulin in type 1 DM affect the process you described in question 3?

5. What are the four basic signs of hyperglycemia? Define them.

a.

b.

c.

d.

CD-ROM Activity

Take the elevator to the Pediatric Unit (Floor 3). Once there, log in to see Jason Baker in Room 306 at 05:30. Jason is a 14-year-old boy who was diagnosed with type 1 diabetes mellitus at the age of 5 years. He is now in the hospital because of a leg fracture. Listen to the Case Overview and click on the **Assignment** to get preliminary information about Jason. Go to his Patient Records and select his Chart. Read his History & Physical, Nursing History, Admission Records, Physician Orders, Progress Notes, and Laboratory Reports related to his insulin, lab tests, and glucose testing. Use the space below and on the next page to write down important points.

Student Notes—Jason Baker

Case Overview and Assignment

History & Physical

Nursing History

Admission Records

Physician Orders—Medications

Progress Notes

Laboratory Reports

6. What are the results of Jason's urine testing?

7. What should the nurse do about the lack of a urine test?

8. What nursing assessment findings relate to Jason's diabetes?

9. How do the assessment and analysis of Jason differ from the usual clinical picture of a person with type 1 diabetes mellitus?

10. The physician has ordered Jason to have fingerstick glucose monitoring a.c. and h.s. Describe the procedures for obtaining a fingerstick blood glucose. (*Hint:* You may need to refer to your own nursing procedures book to answer this question.)

11. What is the normal level of blood glucose for an adolescent?

12. Why are synthetic human insulins (Humulin) recommended for children with type 1 diabetes mellitus?

Go to your pharmacology textbook and review the two insulin medications that Jason is receiving.

 Return to the Nurses' Station and review the MAR for Jason's specific medication orders.

13. Write a medication information summary for the two insulins listed below.

	Regular Insulin	NPH Insulin
Action		
Onset		
Peak		
Duration		
Side effects		
Nursing implications		

14. What are the insulin orders for Jason, as documented in his MAR?

15. Why does Jason receive two different types (strengths) of insulin?

16. Printed below is a chart of insulin action by time. Circle the information you will need to apply to Jason.

Insulin Action by Type (Humulin)			
Type	**Onset**	**Peak**	**Duration**
Lispro	15-30 min	60-90 min	2-3 hr
Regular	30 min	2-4 hr	4-6 hr
NPH or Lente	2-4 hr	6-8 hr	12-24 hr
Ultralente	>2 hr	Variable	24-36 hr

17. Jason is receiving regular and NPH insulin morning and night. Indicate on the timeline below the peak (mark with a P) and duration (use a highlighter to shade this) of his daily insulin doses based on when he receives each dose.

Regular insulin

| 06:30 | 09:00 | 11:00 | 13:00 | 15:00 | 17:00 | 19:00 | Time |

NPH insulin

18. Based on your answers to question 17, when would you most likely expect Jason to have a reaction? Why?

19. Describe the procedure for drawing up regular and NPH insulin into a syringe.

20. What is the correct technique for giving Jason his insulin? Describe the procedure.

21. Rotation of insulin injection sites is important. Why?

22. On the figure below, mark with an X the placement of the 06:30 insulin injection Jason received in the hospital. (Since this was not charted, choose the best site.)

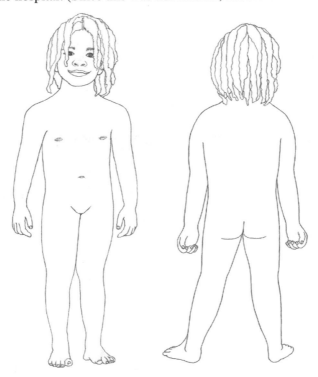

23. What site will you use for Jason's next insulin injection? Circle it on the figure above.

24. Why do Jason's orders have a sliding scale order related to insulin dosage based on blood glucose levels?

25. In the chart below, record Jason's blood glucose readings since admission and assess the trend.

Time	Blood Glucose Reading	Trend

➡ Return to Jason's Chart and click on **Consults**. Review his diabetic consult.

26. How will these recommendations change during Jason's home care?

27. How has Jason tried in the past to control his glucose levels? How did this work?

As you begin to plan for Jason's hospital discharge, review the nursing care plan on pp. 931-934 of your textbook, "The Child with Type 1 Diabetes Mellitus in the Community."

28. Below, personalize the care plan for Jason, using each of the listed nursing diagnoses. From the Nurses' Station, click on **Planning Care**, **Setting Priorities**, and **Nursing Care Matrix**. Once you select the appropriate nursing diagnosis, click on **Outcomes & Interventions** to help you complete the table. If you prefer, you can use the lists of NANDA Nursing Diagnoses in Appendix A of your textbook on pp. 1060-1061.

Nursing Diagnosis	Patient Outcomes	Nursing Interventions
Risk for Imbalanced Nutrition: Less Than Body Requirements related to . . .		
Deficient Knowledge About Diabetes Mellitus related to . . .		
Risk for Injury related to . . .		

29. Jason has been giving himself insulin at home. What questions should you ask him related to his at-home administration?

    a.

    b.

    c.

    d.

30. Based on your knowledge about exercise in children with diabetes, what recommendations would you make regarding Jason's diet once he resumes playing sports?

31. For discharge planning, your clinical instructor has asked you to review the differences between hypoglycemia and hyperglycemia with Jason. In the table below, outline the content you plan to go over with Jason.

	Hypoglycemia	Hyperglycemia
Signs		
Causes		
Treatment		

32. Jason tells you that his friends called him and said that they're planning a welcome home party for him. Provide a nursing diagnosis, patient outcomes, and nursing interventions for Jason relating to this postdischarge party, specifically pertaining to the foods he is allowed to eat at the party.

Nursing Diagnosis	Patient Outcomes	Nursing Interventions

33. As part of the discharge plan, you want to give Jason and his family a brochure reminding them about the signs of serious complications. Develop a brochure below. Be sure to cover the potential complications of diabetic ketoacidosis (DKA).

34. What is the cause of diabetic ketoacidosis (DKA)?

35. Describe the usual nursing assessment findings in a person exhibiting DKA.

36. Describe how the nurse can monitor Jason so that he does not exhibit DKA after his surgery.

37. Because Jason is healing from the leg fracture and surgery, what special nursing assessments must you make related to his diabetes?

38. How does diabetes mellitus affect Jason's developmental status?

39. Jason tells you that he made a lot of friends with children who also had diabetes when he went to diabetes summer camp 6 years ago. Now that he's older, he wants to "surf the Net" to learn more about diabetes and to meet others with diabetes. To help him find some appropriate websites, go to Appendix I: Resources For Health Care Providers and Families (pp. 1093-1100 in your textbook) and select three organizations from the available websites. Go to those websites using the web browser of your choice and summarize them below.

Organization	Website	Services Available

a.

b.

c.

LESSON **19** ————————————————

Nursing Grand Rounds— Neuman Systems Model Nursing Process Format

---

Reading Assignment: Foundations of Child Health Nursing (Chapter 1)
Family-Centered Nursing Care (Chapter 2)
Communicating with Children and Families (Chapter 3)
Health Promotion for the Developing Child (Chapter 4)
Health Promotion for the Adolescent (Chapter 9)
The Ill Child in the Hospital and Other Settings (Chapter 12)
Principles and Procedures for Nursing Care of Children
    (Chapter 14)
Pain Management for Children (Chapter 16)
The Child with a Musculoskeletal Alteration (Chapter 27)
Caring for the Child with an Endocrine or Metabolic Alteration
    (Chapter 28)

Patient: Jason Baker, 14 years, Pediatric Unit, Room 306

This optional lesson gives you the opportunity to use the Neuman Systems Model Nursing Process Format to frame a Nursing Grand Rounds presentation of Jason Baker. Application of Betty Neuman's conceptual model (Neuman, 1995, 1996; Neuman et al, 1997) provides the basis for a comprehensive clinical experience with an adolescent patient. Jason's multiple health stressors impact him to the degree that a thorough exploration of his experience provides you with opportunities to use prevention as part of nursing intervention.

Objectives

Upon completion of this lesson, you will be able to:

1. Analyze the stressors affecting an injured adolescent.
2. Synthesize nursing care for an adolescent by using the Neuman Systems Model Nursing Process Format.
3. Develop a Nursing Grand Rounds presentation pertaining to an injured adolescent.

Note: Throughout this lesson you need to be familiar with information regarding Jason's developmental status as an adolescent, as well as his leg fracture and his diabetes mellitus. It is highly recommended that you review all of the content in the textbook that pertains to him prior to beginning this lesson. Pages of probable interest include the following: 6-10, 12-17, 22-24, 30-36, 39-46, 55-61, 67-69, 71-74, 204-222, 306-314, 359-361, 391-393, 421-433, 855-856, 859-862, 874-878, and 922-938.

CD-ROM Activity

You have been asked to give a presentation about Jason Baker, age 14 years, in this week's Nursing Grand Rounds. To do so, you have decided to frame your presentation using Betty Neuman's Systems Model. First, review the Neuman Systems Model and its components by reading the textbook of your choice to learn about the model. You can also refresh your memory by glancing through the Neuman format used in this lesson. Once you are familiar with the type of information you need to gather about Jason, you will be ready to visit him.

Click **Floor 3** on the elevator selection pad. Go to the Nurses' Station and log in in to visit Jason Baker at 05:30 in Room 306. Remember, Jason has diabetes and he had surgery to reduce a fractured right tibia/fibula. Observe his Preoperative Interview and review his Patient Records. Also click on **Patient Care** and review all sections of information available on Jason's health status.

Then jump ahead in virtual time to when Jason has returned to the Pediatric Floor from surgery (11:00). To do this, you must return to the Nurses' Station, log out on the Supervisor's Computer, and then return to the Nurses' Station to log in for Jason at 11:00. Review his updated Patient Records and then click on **Patient Care** to visit him in his room. At all times, remember to wash your hands when entering and leaving his room.

Once you have thoroughly familiarized yourself with Jason, prepare your presentation by completing the questions in this lesson. In order to complete the process successfully, make sure that you refer frequently to the appropriate pages in your textbook.

1. Begin by briefly summarizing the Neuman Systems Model.

2. Describe each of the following components of Neuman's model, using Jason as the client system, in order to plan the Prevention as Intervention (Primary, Secondary, and Tertiary) for Jason.

NURSING DIAGNOSIS:

DATABASE

PERSON

Client/Client System

    Individual–

    Family–

    Community–

    Social Issue–

Interacting Variables

    Physiological Variable–

    Psychological Variable–

    Sociocultural Variable–

    Developmental Variable–

    Spiritual Variable–

Central Core–

Flexible Line of Defense–

Normal Line of Defense–

Lines of Resistance–

ENVIRONMENT

Internal Environment–

External Environment–

Created Environment–

Stressors

Intrapersonal Stressors–

Interpersonal Stressors–

Extrapersonal Stressors–

ACTUAL VARIANCES FROM WELLNESS

POTENTIAL VARIANCES FROM WELLNESS

NURSING GOALS:

NURSING OUTCOMES:

PRIMARY PREVENTION AS INTERVENTION

SECONDARY PREVENTION AS INTERVENTION

TERTIARY PREVENTION AS INTERVENTION

3. Outline your Nursing Grand Rounds presentation in the space below.

References

Aylward PD: Betty Neuman: The Neuman Systems Model and Global Applications. In Parker M, editor: *Nursing Theories and Nursing Practice*, Philadelphia, 2001, FA Davis, pp 329-342.

Fawcett J: *Analysis and Evaluation of Contemporary Nursing Knowledge: Nursing Models and Theories*, Philadelphia, 2000, FA Davis.

Neuman B: *The Neuman Systems Model*, ed 3, Norwalk, CT, 1995, Appleton & Lange.

Neuman B: The Neuman Systems Model in Research and Practice, *Nursing Science Quarterly* 9:67-70, 1996.

Neuman B, Chadwick PL, Beynon CE, Craig DM, Fawcett J, Chang NJ, Freeze BT, Hinton-Walker P: The Neuman Systems Model: Reflections and Projections, *Nursing Science Quarterly* 10:18-21, 1997.

LESSON 20

Discharge Planning and Health Teaching for Children and Parents: Health Teaching Tool Versus Roy Adaptation Model Tool

Reading Assignment: Health Promotion for the Developing Child (Chapter 4)
Health Promotion for the School-Age Child (Chapter 8)
The Child with a Chronic Condition or Terminal Illness
(Chapter 13)
The Child with a Respiratory Disorder (Chapter 22)
The Child with Cancer (Chapter 25)
Resources for Health Care Providers and Families (Appendix I)

Patients: De Olp, 6 years old, Pediatric Unit, Room 310
Maria Ortiz, 8 years old, Pediatric Unit, Room 308

Synthesis of health care for children and families at home and in the community is the focus of this lesson. Here you will develop and pilot-test two discharge planning tools. One is a standard health teaching tool, and the other is a tool based on the Roy Adaptation Model (Roy & Andrews, 1999; Roy & Zhan, 2001). In these cases, you will use your comprehensive knowledge about two school-age girls who have long-term health care needs. The patients are De Olp, a 6-year-old girl diagnosed with acute lymphocytic leukemia, and 8-year-old Maria Ortiz, who has asthma. This culminating virtual clinical experience encourages you to use your own critical thinking skills to plan discharge needs for children and families.

Objectives

Upon completion of this lesson, you will be able to:

1. Analyze long-term health needs for two children with chronic illnesses.
2. Develop and pilot-test discharge planning tools for school-age children.
3. Anticipate health teaching for children living at home with long-term illnesses.
4. Synthesize nursing care based on the Roy Adaptation Model.

 Go to your textbook and review sections in the following chapters that relate to the school-age child and chronic illness:
  Chapter 4, Health Promotion for the Developing Child
  Chapter 8, Health Promotion for the School-Age Child
  Chapter 13, The Child with a Chronic Condition or Terminal Illness

Next, review the nursing care for the child with leukemia and the child with asthma in the following chapters:
  Chapter 22, The Child with a Respiratory Disorder
  Chapter 25, The Child with Cancer

The discharge planning nurse has asked you to pilot-test two health teaching guides for children and families who will need a long period of health maintenance at home. You are aware that there are two such children and families familiar to you in the Pediatric Unit of Canyon View Regional Medical Center: De Olp (6 years old) and Maria Ortiz (8 years old). You decide to use these children's needs as a pattern to help you test the forms. De's needs are outlined on the standard form; Maria's on the Roy form.

CD-ROM Activity

Take the elevator to the Pediatric Unit (Floor 3). At the Nurses' Station, log in to visit De Olp, age 6 years, at 07:00 in Room 310. After watching the Case Overview, return to the Nurses' Station, click on **Patient Records** and review any sections of De's Chart you wish. Visit De in her room by clicking **Patient Care** and **Data Collection**. Remember to wash your hands before entering her room. Observe any sections of the physical assessment that will help you with your planning. After your visit, make an assessment of De's home discharge needs and what she and her parents may need to be taught to facilitate health teaching.

1. For each category in the Home Discharge Planning Tool below and on the next page, fill in the patient teaching information required for De and her parents.

HOME DISCHARGE PLANNING TOOL

Categories for Discharge Planning	De Olp
Home Routines	
Potential for Infection and Vaccinations	
Nutrition	
Medications	
At Home	
At School	

School-Related Needs

Recreation

Schedule for Follow-Up
Appointments

Referrals Needed

Community Resources

Future Plans

→ Since you need to gather health information about Maria Ortiz as well, log out from seeing De by returning to the Nurses' Station and clicking on the Supervisor's Computer. Then return to the Nurses' Station again and log in to visit Maria Ortiz at 07:00 in Room 308. Review her Patient Records and observe the Data Collection as needed to learn about Maria's health care needs. (Wash your hands!)

2. To begin planning Maria's discharge needs, you first need to complete an assessment of her behavior. Fill out the sections below and on the next page that relate to Maria.

ROY ADAPTATION MODEL NURSING PROCESS for Maria Ortiz

ASSESSMENT OF BEHAVIOR

Physiological/Physical Mode

Oxygenation

Nutrition

Elimination

Activity & Rest

Protection

Senses

Fluid, Electrolytes & Acid-Base Balance

Neurological Function

Endocrine Function

Self-Concept Mode

Physical Self

Personal Self

Role Function Mode

Primary Role

Secondary Role

Tertiary Role

Interdependence Mode

Developmental Adequacy

3. Now that you have organized the data needed to plan for Maria's discharge, continue using the Roy format to define Maria's health teaching needs.

Assessment of Stimuli	Nursing Diagnosis (NANDA)	Goal Setting	Health Teaching Interventions	Evaluation
Focal Stimuli				
Contextual Stimuli				
Residual Stimuli				

4. Compare and contrast the discharge needs of De and Maria. Are they similar or different? Provide a rationale for your answer.

References

Fawcett J: *Analysis and Evaluation of Contemporary Nursing Knowledge: Nursing Models and Theories*, Philadelphia, 2000, FA Davis.

Roy C, Andrews HA: *The Roy Adaptation Model*, ed 2, Stamford, CT, 1999, Appleton & Lange.

Roy C, Zhan L: Sister Callista Roy: The Roy Adaptation Model. In Parker M, *Nursing Theories and Nursing Practice*, Philadelphia, 2001, FA Davis, pp 315-328.